THE CHILD–PARENT CAREGIVING RELATIONSHIP IN LATER LIFE

Psychosocial Experiences

Bethany Morgan Brett

First published in Great Britain in 2023 by

Policy Press, an imprint of
Bristol University Press
University of Bristol
1–9 Old Park Hill
Bristol
BS2 8BB
UK
t: +44 (0)117 374 6645
e: bup-info@bristol.ac.uk

Details of international sales and distribution partners are available at
policy.bristoluniversitypress.co.uk

British Library Cataloguing in Publication Data
A catalogue record for this book is available from the British Library

ISBN 978-1-4473-1929-0 hardcover
ISBN 978-1-4473-1969-6 paperback
ISBN 978-1-4473-2431-7 ePub
ISBN 978-1-4473-1970-2 ePdf

The right of Bethany Morgan Brett to be identified as author of this work has been asserted by her in
accordance with the Copyright, Designs and Patents Act 1988.

Cover design: Robin Hawes
Front cover image: iStock/WoodenheadWorld
Bristol University Press and Policy Press use environmentally responsible
print partners.
Printed and bound in Great Britain by CPI Group (UK) Ltd, Croydon, CR0 4YY

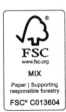

FSC
www.fsc.org
MIX
Paper | Supporting
responsible forestry
FSC® C013604

For all our parents

Contents

Acknowledgements

My first acknowledgement of thanks must go to all those people who shared their intimate stories of their lives and relationships. Thanks to the people living and working in care homes across Essex who allowed me to spend time with them, listen to their life stories, and to observe their lives in care. Thank you to My Home Life England (staff and volunteers) for facilitating access to the care homes and for all the transformational work you are doing to improve the quality of life for older people in residential care.

My second acknowledgement of thanks goes to three inspiring academics. First, the late Professor Ian Craib, who encouraged me to explore psychoanalysis and how it could be incorporated into sociology, developing a psychosocial approach. Ian also first encouraged me into researching the academic topics of ageing, death, dying, loss, and the importance of disappointment. Second, Professor Mike Roper, who supported me through my PhD journey and our discussions were always challenging and thought-provoking. And third, Chris Tanner, who has always been a huge support to me, championed my research, and was a co-researcher on the two My Home Life England evaluations. I am also grateful for the funding from the ESRC, Joseph Rowntree Fund, Essex County Council, and from the University of East London's Early Career Accelerator Grant, which have supported the various stages of this research.

I would like to especially thank my husband Bryan for his endless support, patience, love, encouragement, and for always keeping me grounded. Thank you to my parents Janice and the late Neil, to my late parents-in-law Janet and Malcolm for all the support over the years, and to my sister Bryony, who is the epitome of strength and determination.

Thank you to the editors and the publication team at Policy Press for their unwavering support patience and motivation for me on this project and to the anonymous reviewers for their encouraging and constructive feedback on earlier drafts. This book has been written during some trying times including my own serious illness, my husband's serious illness, the death of three of our four parents, and not to mention a global pandemic! It has not been easy and has taken much longer than I had anticipated, but I believe firmly in growing through adversity. Each of these huge life experiences has brought with it new insight which has contributed to the writing of this book.

Introduction

Hazel

When I arrived to interview Hazel[1] at her North London home, I found that she had prepared my favourite lunch. We had never met before, but she had secretively asked our mutual contact what I might like. She showed me around her home and even offered me a pair of guest slippers to wear, an invitation perhaps, to 'take a walk in her shoes'. This visit became more than an interview; instead it was a day of sharing intimate stories of profoundly difficult experiences surrounding the changing relationship she had had with her mother in the final years of her life.

Towards the end of the day, Hazel showed me her family documents. As she flicked through the digital photographs on her desk-top computer she skipped past one rather quickly. I asked if she would mind going back, as that photograph had caught my attention. "Oh," she said, "that's not a good picture. I am crying in that one." "Would you mind telling me about the story behind that photo?" I asked. She told me that this was a photo taken at her mother's 100th birthday party and that the day had been particularly difficult.

'[The 100th birthday] was a turning point in all ways. One, you know, she was a hundred, how extraordinary! And two, that was when she went into care. She went in just a few days later. And actually, I don't regret it. I didn't regret it at the time. I don't regret it now, at all. It's a step, isn't it? And I can't, I can't work out why it's so difficult', Hazel said with tears pricking in her eyes. 'It's a loss – excuse me. It's a loss, but erm, it's also an incredible gain. It was a gain for me, because I was feeling that a lot of my life was getting lost in terms of where my energy was going. I was losing, I was losing, I was losing touch with people. I mean, everybody would ask after her, and lots of people came with me to see her. My friend Jonah came fairly regularly; Paul came from Thailand, you know. Erm, people would come with me to see her, and Josie came every week, for God's sake, you know! But I felt my energy was being sapped by all of this. Does that make sense?'

'Absolutely, yes.'

'Well, it doesn't matter if it doesn't make sense, because that's how it feels,' she said kindly. 'And there's, something else, erm, I'm trying to feel for. Well, I lost my mum. That's it. I mean, I'd have lost her

---

[1] All names of participants have been changed to protect their identities.

when she died, anyway, but Alzheimer's is so cruel because there's the person, and there's, I'm not saying there's nothing in there, of course there is, but it doesn't come out. In the end, I don't think Mum knew her name. But she did used to say umm – well I'm glad she didn't live much longer, because if she'd forgotten who I was, I don't know what I would have done.'

'So, she recognised who *you were*, but she didn't recognise *her* own name?' I clarified.

Hazel nodded and replied tearfully, 'She'd say, "There's my baby".'

★★★

This book presents the intimate stories of changing relationships between adult children and their ageing parents in the caregiving role in later life. Its aim is to offer new insights into the physical, emotional, and psychical effects the witnessing of increasing agedness and loss of parents has on the adult child, and to highlight the emotional complexity of making decisions of care for and with older parents.

Drawing upon data collected across five distinct qualitative and literature-based research projects, this book travels through the stages of the relationship with an older parent who requires care in the later stages of life.

We will hear the voices of adult children and how they began identifying and managing the care needs of their older parents at home. Their stories highlight the emotional impact of caregiving and how roles, responsibilities, and dynamics shift within the family when older parents require care. We will hear the stories of how decisions have been made for and with older parents to transition into residential social care provision, as well as hearing the narratives of older people living in care and what life is now like for them. Towards the end of the book, we will look at the psychological experience of losing a parent in later life, not just through a final biological death but the commonly preceding losses associated with cognitive decline.

This book highlights how the social experiences and cultural expectations, which surround the care for a parent in later life, also influence the adult child's attitudes and pragmatic reactions to ageing, and these are necessarily intertwined with unconscious psychic processes, conflicts, and ambivalence. There has been significant research conducted on the experience of older people living in care, and on instrumental care tasks, but there is surprisingly little written on the adult child's psychological experience of a changing relationship with their parent as they age. Adult children are often intrinsically bound with the decision-making and transition to care processes, and this has a significant impact on their lives. It will be argued that witnessing the ageing of a parent in later life can be extremely stressful, unsettling, and emotionally complex.

Difficult decisions have to be made for increasingly dependent parents (Umberson, 2003). The loss of a parent (as you know them and/or through death) and the consequent grief and mourning that follows evokes a series of complicated psychological challenges, and sees a realignment of family roles and dynamics as the generational family tree shifts. There can be a complex mix of conflicting emotions for the adult child, including an increased sense of responsibility, maturity, and wisdom, to feelings of vulnerability, anger, grief, loss, and anxiety, as the relationship with their older parent is forever changed.

The older parent and the adult child

Throughout this book I will use the terms 'adult child' and 'older parent' quite deliberately. Firstly, I am avoiding the simpler term of 'parent' as I want to convey here the specificity to parents in the later stages of life. Secondly, I am using the term 'older parent' in favour of the term 'elderly parent'. Often older people experience negative stereotypes and harmful attitudes towards them based on their age, and ageist discrimination is often presented through the way that language is used to describe this age group (Amundsen, 2022). 'The term *elderly* is ageist' (Avers et al, 2011) and tends to convey stereotypes of vulnerability, dependency, loneliness, and marginalisation (Amundsen, 2022), whereas the term 'older adult', or 'older parent', as is used here, is intended to convey a wider spectrum of experience. Even where the older parent described in this book may be in a position of vulnerability and dependency, they still have opportunity for self-expression, inclusivity, autonomy, and agency.

I use the term 'adult child' in a considered way too, and here I am referring specifically to an adult who has a parent in later life. I am using this term in favour of 'family member', or 'informal caregiver' as I specifically want to focus on the child–parent relationship, which may or may not involve elements of caregiving. As you will read later in this book, some adult children were reluctant to engage in caregiving activities for their parents, and some were reluctant to have their role title changed from 'son' or 'daughter' to 'carer' as their parent aged. Also, I felt that the term 'adult child' conveyed something of the inner psychological experience of relating to a parent in later life. The majority of adult children who have parents in the later stages of life are in the mid- or late midlife stages of the life course. This is a life stage characterised by significant changes in personal circumstances, and although many of these changes are anticipated, their impact can still come as a surprise, reawakening old psychological threats, anxieties, and defences which were first experienced in the early infantile stages such as the psychological conflicts surrounding loss, guilt, frustration, abandonment, separation, and attachment.

The ageing population

Life expectancy worldwide is increasing due to overall improved medical innovations, better nutrition, and improvements in working and living conditions (Seidlein et al, 2018). Worldwide, countries are faced with the challenge of providing health and social care to their ageing populations (Barron and West, 2017). The UK is no exception with a population of 11 million people aged over 65 (Office for National Statistics, 2022) with that figure set to increase to almost 13 million in the next 10 years (Centre for Ageing Better, 2022). Amongst the older population there are over 600,000 (Office for National Statistics, 2021b) people aged 90+ and there are over 15,000 are centenarians (Office for National Statistics, 2021b).

People are increasingly living to what Neugarten (1974) termed 'old old age', Laslett (1989) called 'the fourth age', and what Featherstone and Hepworth (1989) labelled 'deep old age'. However, whilst longevity is often celebrated, advancing age is often accompanied by ongoing ill-health and disabilities which require the support from others to assist older adults in their daily living. The number of years of life expected to be spent without a disability or in good health is referred to as a 'healthy life expectancy' (Office for National Statistics, 2018). Yet it is important to note that life expectancy is rising more quickly than healthy life expectancy, meaning more people are living longer but in poorer health.

As the number of people with complex care needs increases in the UK population, society is challenged by how they are to be cared for, resulting in an increased demand for informal and formal long-term care (Gans et al, 2009). However, there have been significant (and 'rapidly deteriorating' (Bath, 2017)) political, societal, and economic changes in recent years, and this includes increased demands upon health-care systems and cuts to public resources. The National Health Service is simultaneously under-resourced and experiencing unprecedented high demand, particularly since the coronavirus pandemic which was declared in March 2020. Increasing demands upon care systems in combination with public spending cuts means that without drastic government intervention formal long-term care will only be available to the very oldest in society and informal caregiving will increase.

Currently, informal family caregivers provide the majority of long-term care for older parents. Achenbaum (2005, p 25) writes that 'family members have always been the primary line of defence in situations of old-age dependency'. Along with these expanding responsibilities for adult children in midlife there have been concurrent changes in familial structures which have an impact on care provision for older family members. For instance, increasing rates of divorce and reconstituted family arrangements have put families under 'considerable risk of disruption and strain in intergenerational bonds' (Gans et al, 2009, p 404). Informal caregiving can have a significant effect on the adult child's quality of life, impacting them physically, emotionally, and financially. However, much of this informal caregiving remains hidden, and unacknowledged by society and health-care systems (Seidlein et al, 2018). Furthermore, a move into a caregiving role for an older parent can often be unexpected and confronting, inducing caregiving role strain, as the adult child is thrust into a role where they have not developed the skills necessary for such a position. One of the primary reasons an older person is moved into long-term care is due to a change in the capacity of the carer to care for them. Sometimes this follows a spousal death in later life, someone who up until that point had been an at-home support for the older person. Care provision for an older parent becomes increasingly demanding as their frailty increases, and the caregiving burden of adult children is not only associated with lower well-being scores for them, but also for their older parent (Lewis, 2014, p 1222). Brodaty and Donkin (2009, p 217) write that 'family caregivers of people with dementia, often called the invisible second patients, are critical to the quality of life of the care recipients', and whilst significant scholarly activity has been undertaken to explore the experiences of older people, far less attention has been paid to the experiences of their adult children upon which many older people are dependent for a good quality of life.

The crisis of care

Widening health and wealth inequalities have a significant impact upon not only how long we live and in what level of health, but also upon the experiences of caregiving and care receiving. There is an increasing disparity in wealth and income among people in their 50s and 60s, which has seen the 'the net (non-pension) wealth of the richest 20% of people in this age group doubled between 2002 and 2018, while that of the poorest 20% fell by 30%' (The Centre for Ageing Better, 2022, p 8). This socio-economic disparity impacts on the care arrangements for older people in that those in socially and economically disadvantaged positions are more likely to provide informal caregiving for older family members and 'end up trapped in caring roles with even fewer labour market opportunities and thus find themselves at higher risk of poverty' (Naiditch et al, 2013, p 59). Whereas, in contrast, those with a higher socio-economic status have the resources to outsource their care responsibilities. 'Arber and Ginn (1993) note that the resources possessed by the middle class enable them to care "at a distance" while working class people, with fewer available options, are more likely to provide informal care within the household' (Chappell and Penning, 2005, p 458).

Whilst in the UK health care is free at the point of use in the National Health Service (NHS), state support for adult social care is means tested. This can come as a surprise to some adult children who are seeking care support for their parents, and some assume it is free on the NHS (Franklin, 2015, p 4). There has been a 'long-standing debate' about who should bear the cost of care (Lloyd, 2012, p 3) and whether this should be borne by the individual or the state. Lloyd (2012, p 3) acknowledges that 'in the context of population ageing at a time of dominant neoliberal economic policies the terms of the debate have been changed and the question increasingly is not whether but *how* and *to what* extent individuals should bear the cost' (emphasis in original text). Local authorities have some responsibility for co-funding adult social care services, if the care recipient cannot afford to meet their care needs (Simpson, 2017). However, due to spending cuts there has been a fall in public expenditure on adult social care in recent years (Franklin, 2015, p 4). Local authority budgets have been under pressure due to demographic changes, the number of older people accessing social care, increases in the National Living Wage, which have placed additional costs upon local councils to pay care staff a fair wage, and most significantly over the last two years, the COVID-19 pandemic has created enormous funding pressures (Foster, 2023, p 5). Foster (2023, p 9) writes that 'estimates of the size of the social care "funding gap" vary', but that in 2020 the Health and Social Care Committee said in their report that 'an additional £7bn per year was required by 2023/24'.

The impact of COVID-19

In January 2020 the World Health Organisation (WHO) declared COVID-19 a public health emergency of international concern, formally declaring it a pandemic in March 2020. The UK government's response was to test, track, and trace, acquire additional personal protective equipment (PPE), restrict all unnecessary social interactions, and impose a series of strict lockdowns. This had a significant impact on many people's physical and mental health, had a drastic impact upon the economy, and a devastating effect on the lives of those living, working, and dying in social care settings.

The health risks and associated restrictions created a particular strain on family relationships and caregiving responsibilities. There were changes in routine and adult children frequently had to juggle multiple responsibilities including working from home, whilst caring for children and grandchildren (and home-schooling) and looking after older relatives – sometimes all within the same household. Some people lost their jobs and many people worried about their household or business finances. In addition, many of the external care support services such as day centres or respite services, which may have helped balance the caregiving burden pre-pandemic, were reduced or even withdrawn during this period.

For those families whose older relatives were living in care homes, the pandemic was equally as challenging. The majority of access to care homes was restricted, even to the closest of relatives, due to the significant health risks the virus posed. The spread of COVID-19 was of particular concern in care home settings due to the close living conditions of residents, many of whom are living with health vulnerabilities and co-morbidities. 'Care home residents accounted for 33% of all COVID-19 related deaths in England' (Comas-Herrera et al, 2020, p 16). Hudson (2021, p 121) reported that there were estimates of over 20,000 deaths in care homes, and care home occupancy rates declined to around 80 per cent, which threatened many homes with financial collapse. And even *within* care homes there was isolation, with residents being segregated and quarantined for fear of outbreaks, meaning that some residents were confined to their rooms (Lightfoot and Moone, 2020), which only increased older peoples' experience of seclusion and loneliness during this period. Lightfoot and Moone's (2020) study into the impact of the COVID-19 pandemic on caregiving showed that families whose relatives lived in care during the pandemic faced a number of challenges. Relatives were unable to visit the care home for long periods of time, which was particularly distressing if their older parent did not understand what was happening or why they were not able to visit. Families became increasingly concerned about the health of their older relative, who was at a higher risk of infection from the virus by virtue of their advancing age, their proximity to other older people living in the close environment of a care home, and higher mortality risks if they did catch it. Family caregivers worried about becoming infected with COVID-19 themselves and passing it on to their vulnerable older loved ones. Lightfoot and Moone (2020) highlighted the sense of helplessness that relatives felt when they could not protect their family members or provide the type or amount of care that they would usually want to provide. The long-term emotional consequences, or trauma, of COVID-19, as yet remain unknown.

The pandemic further highlighted the systematic inadequacies of the current social care system (Age UK, Health and Care Bill, 2022), forcing adult social care into public awareness. One element of the system that was particularly highlighted was the vital role of care staff (arguably signified by the 'clap for carers' movement) and a new appreciation for care roles, as many put their own health at risk during this period caring for others. Yet, at the same time, it was also revealed how precarious care worker employment is, with an increasing proportion of staff on undervalued and underpaid casualised contracts.

The data collection period for the research upon which this book is based was accomplished before the COVID-19 pandemic and, as such, there is only a limited reflection upon the impact of the pandemic on care relationships. However, I do recognise that further research in this area is needed, and is indeed already emerging (see Hudson, 2021; Lightfoot and Moone, 2020; and The Care Collective, 2020).

Chapter summaries

This book's perspective is primarily from the psychosocial experience of the adult child, and it is therefore these voices which are prioritised. It explores how decisions of care are made for and with their older parents and how their relationship is navigated during this process. However, we will hear older people's voices more prominently in Chapter 4, 'Materiality, clothing, and embodiment in care', and Chapter 5, 'Social connections and relationship building in residential care'.

A disclaimer: At this stage I should offer an explanation as to what this book is and what it is not. Whilst there is some discussion about how a care home is chosen, and what life in care is like from the perspective of the older adult, this book is not intended as a self-help text, nor is it a guide to choosing care provision. I also now work for My Home Life England and recognise the tremendous work that they do, and although some of my research was conducted simultaneously with previous evaluation work for My Home Life England the views and opinions contained in this book are my own and have been collated from many years of independent research in this field. Please see Appendix 1, 'Researching the child–parent caregiving relationship', for the full details of the research journey.

This is a book which raises the voices of an under-represented population of adult child relatives who care for their older parents. Its aim is to highlight the significant impact a caring role has on the adult child, and how this is intertwined with unconscious psychic processes. It is hoped that it will encourage social policy changes by offering a more focused consideration of the emotional experiences of the adult child whilst they witness and care for ageing parents. Its aim it to promote new ways of thinking about care and relationship, particularly in the distinct midlife period of the life course.

The chapters of this book are framed around a transitional journey from recognising that a parent requires care, to moving into care, to settling into life in a care home, and to recognising and coming to terms with the loss of parents in later life.

Chapter 1, 'Midlife and the adult child', sets the theoretical scene around themes of ageing and midlife. It presents a critical look at the life course, with particular focus on Erikson's (1950) psychosocial stage model which outlines some of the challenges faced in the mid to latter part of the life course. One such challenge is the 'generational shift', which sees the upward movement of the generations, and for those in midlife, places them higher up in the hierarchy of the family tree. This can have consequences for the way in which the adult child experiences their own ageing, and how family roles and relationships are negotiated.

This generational shift, and the witnessing of a parent's ageing process, brings the midlife individual's own sense of ageing to the fore, resulting in increased existential anxiety. This existential anxiety has consequences for the way in which midlife children experience their own ageing process and has an impact on their relationships with their older parents.

Chapter 2, 'Becoming a carer', focuses on how family relationships can change when making decisions about care for an ageing parent. In particular, historic tensions within sibling dynamics, which perhaps have been put aside or ignored as they have grown older, are reignited when pushed together to make decisions for parents (Khodyakov and Carr, 2009). There is sometimes uncertainty about who should perform which role or task within a family system, once the 'leader' or figurehead of the parent is incapacitated or dies. There will be illustrations of both coordination and a clear division of labour amongst cooperative groups of siblings as well as complete breakdowns of relationships in some families. In addition, Chapter 2 will look at the experience of the 'only child' and how they often have more autonomy about care choices and have more say on what happens to property and possessions. Only children reported increased bonds with parents, but also sometimes felt a little lonely in their situations due to a lack of social and emotional support.

The final part of this chapter looks at the experiences of adult children when first faced with a parent whose health has deteriorated. If a parent is showing symptoms of onset dementia, the adult child may be challenged by their role and how to relate to their parent. The roles may have suddenly reversed and whereas once they were a son or daughter to their parent, they now find themselves in new roles as a carer or a parent's parent, and this can be deeply unsettling (Umberson and Chen, 1994). Moreover, providing care at home (in a parent's or an adult child's) can be physically and mentally exhausting. Despite valiant efforts from adult children to enable independent living in the older parents' own homes, it was often a huge daily battle and emotional burden, leading to what has become commonly known as 'caregiver burden' (Young et al, 2006). Carrying out physical, intimate tasks for a parent can be a difficult aspect of care provision, but for some it can also be an important bonding experience (Umberson, 2010).

Chapter 3 addresses 'The transition to care'. Although this book will not be focusing on the alternative arrangements for care such as moving in with adult children, or moving to sheltered housing, these options are discussed in conversations between parents and adult children here. The focus of the discussion here is specifically on older parents who have lived in their own homes and now face moving into residential care homes. We take a look at the transition into long-term care and how this topic is first broached within family discussions. Chapter 3 also looks at how, despite careful discussions, arguments, and conflicting opinions about whether a parent should or could go into residential care, in most cases the slow burn of declining health and incremental care duties are often accelerated beyond the control of both the parent and adult child, usually resulting from a fall followed by rapid decline in dementia (Ball et al, 2014).

However, for those who do have to choose a care home for a parent, this is often new territory and a significant practical challenge as well as an emotional one, as being faced with a minefield of choice can be overwhelming and anxiety provoking. The section will consider the emotional and practical challenges faced by the adult child with their older parent when making these decisions.

Chapter 4, 'Materiality, clothing, and embodiment in care', considers the role of objects in the transition into a resident care home. It reflects upon the personal possessions which are taken by the older person into a care home and what these mean to them, and which objects are brought to the home on their behalf. It will consider how objects are chosen, managed, or disposed of in the move to care. It will also look at the adult child's experience of clearing a parent's home.

Managing what happens to a parent's home and possessions is one of the biggest challenges related to care decisions. The rapid decline of a parent's health, often following a fall or other crisis, means that decisions that have been put off are suddenly accelerated in their urgency. In most cases, the transition into care means that the parent's home needs to be sold or rented out, and, in many cases, homes need redecorating or updating to be marketed. There can be an emotional attachment to the home with many of the older people having lived there for their entire adult lives and raising their children there. Often an older parent is the family's anchor, and their home the family's centre. In some cases, the parent's home is also the adult child's childhood home, so issues of sentimentality can hinder the process of clearing or selling the property and make the task emotionally challenging. Moreover, sorting a house of its possessions – choosing which things a parent might like, choosing which items to sell, which to give to charity, which to pass on as heirlooms, which to keep, finding important paperwork, finding all the photographs – is a task which needs to be done, but is time-consuming and exhausting for the adult child who may also be contending with visits to the care home, holding down a job, maintaining their own home, and in some cases still be caring for their own children too. And how they then select personal possessions for someone else requires a great deal of thought and care (Ward et al, 2014; and Buse and Twigg, 2014).

The final part of this chapter looks at the particular significance clothing has in the older person's life. Clothing allows for an expression of self, can maintain connections to past experiences and identities, provide a sense of comfort and safety in the unfamiliar environment of a new care home, and can play a role in connecting with others.

Chapter 5, 'Social connections and relationship building in residential care', highlights some of the challenges faced by older people as they settle into their new home, but also reveals how they find new avenues of self-expression, autonomy, and friendship. Some parent–child relationships grow stronger as they find new ways to connect, now freed from the instrumental care tasks which preceded the move.

In this chapter we will look at the experience of visiting a parent in a care home and how geographical mobility and the use of technology can impact upon the degrees of contact adult children and older parents can have with one another. The chapter also looks at the experiences of relationship building and relationship breakdowns when visiting an older parent in care. In addition to the practical considerations of moving, there is a great depth of emotional response and adult children have a propensity to fall into a cycle of guilt, which occurs when they do not visit for a while because they feel guilty for putting their parent in a home, and then feel even guiltier for not visiting and so stop visits altogether. Some parents do not necessarily even remember a visit, and this can make visits feel pointless and unfulfilling for the adult child.

The final, thematic chapter, Chapter 6, examines 'The loss of parents in later life'. The focus here is less on the period of grief following a death and the practicalities of funeral arrangements, but rather more on the feelings surrounding what Dupuis (2002) called anticipatory or ambiguous loss, which is when those people who feel the death of a loved one is imminent could experience this as an impending loss, which requires mourning before the bereavement itself occurs (Boss, 2012). Finally, in this chapter I explore the ambivalent feelings that are aroused by the death of parents, including feelings of grief, sadness, depression, and guilt, but also relief, opportunity, empowerment, self-development, and freedom.

1

Midlife and the adult child

There has been significant research conducted on the experience of older people living in care but much less written on the experience of adult children who are so often intrinsically bound with the decision-making and transition process. The adult children represented in this book are in the mid- to late-midlife period of the life course and so it is important to consider the psychosocial challenges which impact on this period of the life course.

Midlife signifies an important stage of transition characterised by significant changes in personal circumstances, and although many of these changes are expected their impact can still come as a surprise, reawakening old threats and anxieties and creating new ones. The death of parents, children leaving home, changes at work, awareness of an ageing body – these changes are usually anticipated on a practical level but the emotional and psychological impact that they have can create a sense of instability and insecurity for the midlife adult. In this chapter we will examine some of the theories of the life course with particular focus on the midlife stage. We will see that one particular characterising feature of midlife is an increase in existential anxiety, heightened through an awareness of a generation shift which is, in part, characterised by the ageing and death of older parents.

The life course and its stages

In 1975, sociologist Glen Elder, Jr, distinguished 'life course sociology' as a distinct discipline, based upon five core principles which include (1) *life span development* which recognises that human development is a lifelong process shaped by (2) *historical time and geographical place*, and that (3) *timings* of events in an individual's life are significant. He suggests that human lives are (4) *interlinked* through relationships and shared social networks, and that finally individuals are able to construct their own life course through (5) *agency* but within the framework of opportunities and constraints. Gilleard and Higgs (2016, p 302) later characterised life course sociology in two distinct ways: first, as a series of life stages, each with its own particular set of challenges, obligations, and opportunities, and second as a stratification over the life course in which individual biographies are shaped by historical events, society, and embedded in social institutions.

One of the most well-known models of life span development was established by Erik Erikson and first outlined in his text *Childhood and*

Society (1950). This theory of psychosocial human development proposed that the life course comprises eight distinct sequential, epigenetic stages which lead to the eventual maturation of the individual. Erikson's 'The Eight Ages of Man' include the stages (1) trust vs mistrust, (2) autonomy vs shame and doubt, (3) initiative vs guilt, (4) industry vs inferiority, (5) identity vs confusion, (6) intimacy vs isolation, (7) generativity vs stagnation, and (8) integrity vs despair. Each of Erikson's stages relates to an ego development task and a challenge to be worked through in order to reach a point of fulfilment and integration (Maree, 2021). Each stage builds upon the stages that came before, progressing from birth to old age and death. The model also has a cyclical quality in that if a stage was not completed successfully, it may re-emerge as a challenge again in the future (Zhang, 2015). Influenced by Freud's early work in psychoanalysis, Erikson's model of the life course proposed that early life experiences could influence future personality development. However, whereas Freud's psychoanalytic theory suggested that personality development related primarily to early childhood experiences, Erikson's model developed this further, taking the stages of development into late adolescence, through adulthood and into old age. Erikson's work was particularly innovative in its incorporation of the psychological aspects of human development with the social world, maintaining that they must operate jointly. Hoare (2005, p 19) writes that Erikson revised Freudian thought, shifting it 'upward in consciousness, outward to the social world, and forward throughout the complete life span'.

However, Erikson's model has been challenged by other life course theorists. Drawing on Roazen's (1980) critique, Gilleard and Higgs (2016, p 306) highlight that Erikson's stage model lacks 'critical interrogation of the social context in which adult personality is formed'. Instead, they suggest that individual development is embedded in social institutions, historical events, and cultural context, all of which will affect the way in which an individual might measure success in their lives. Although Erikson was a proponent of the incorporation of the 'psycho' and 'social' aspects of an individual's life, the critical role that institutions play in human development was an area left undeveloped in his theory. For instance, it is important to recognise how someone's social and cultural background – where they live, the community which they are part of, which school they go to, where they work, and in later life which care settings they move to – will significantly impact on their long-term health, well-being, and social development. Furthermore, Erikson was writing in 1950 at a time when life course trajectories and traditional age ordering was more clearly defined. However, shifts in the later part of the twentieth century and into the twenty-first century have seen significant changes in work and the economy, changes in family structures, plasticity of self-identity, and increasingly individualised patterns in social life. All have implications for how the life course is experienced and how caregiving roles are socially contextualised.

Erikson's model has also been criticised for the insufficient attention it pays to the relationships we have with others, particularly when we look at the model through the lens of feminist ethics. The model is inherently gender biased and androcentric, neglecting women's experience of the life course (Gilligan, 1982; Zhang, 2015). A feminist lens on the life course would highlight Elder's (1975) principle of 'linked lives', recognising the importance of shared relationships across the life course, most intimately within the family setting and most critically in a care relationship. Hockey and James (2003) challenged completely Erikson's idea that we have fixed life stages, instead arguing that identity is created and recreated through our interactions with others, through life events, through the passage of time, and ultimately expressed through embodiment.

It is, nevertheless, useful to think about Erikson's framework and the psychological challenges he poses at each stage of the life course. Erikson's model was innovative in building upon Freud's (1905) model of childhood psychosexual development, and advancing description of the stages into early adulthood, midlife, and old age. It is Erikson's latter two stages, (7) generativity vs stagnation and (8) integrity vs despair, which are most interesting for a study on caregiving in later life. The seventh stage maps most closely onto the midlife part of the life course, and the eighth stage onto 'old age'. The psychosocial task of generativity, for example, has significant implications for how meaning in life is created, how legacy is defined, and plays a critical role in managing age-related existential anxiety. This will be explained in more detail as we now discuss the experiences of the midlife adult child and how they relate to their older parents.

Midlife adult children

Midlife as a concept is notoriously difficult to define and the way it has been categorised and re-categorised in the literature has aligned with social, economic, and historical shifts. Over the centuries midlife has been conceptualised as primarily a period of change, loss, and reflection; a juncture between growth and decline (Lachman et al, 2014); a period of crisis and creativity (Jaques, 1965); and a period of generativity or stagnation (Erikson, 1963). One of the first mentions of midlife was by the fourteenth-century poet and philosopher Dante, who at the age of 35 described midlife as wandering lost through a dark forest. In 1965 the psychologist Elliot Jaques described midlife as a crisis point in the life course, occurring at around age 35, which is motivated by an underlying fear of death from which he saw creative impulses arise. Gail Sheehy's *Passages*, published in 1976, also gave a rather pessimistic outlook on the midlife experience but it became one of the best-selling books in America in the 1970s and raised the awareness amongst the general public of midlife as an important life stage. However, there was a shift in the late 1990s to early 2000s, with popular literature and self-help guides writing about *The Middle-Aged Rebel* (Lambley, 1995) and *ReFirement* (Gambone, 2000) as new ways to conceptualise midlife as a more positive, life affirming period of growth.

Earlier accounts of midlife tended to situate midlife in the mid to late thirties whilst the boundaries of later definitions have shifted it to later in the life course as a result of increasing life expectancy. For Jaques, the midlife crisis occurred around the age of 35, but he claimed 'the exact period will vary among individuals' (1965, p 502). However, he was writing in the mid 1960s, and in the UK between 1972 and 1976 the average life expectancy for men from birth was 69.2 years, so midlife would have been 34–35 years old, and for women in 1972–1976 the life expectancy from birth was 75.2, making midlife 37–38. According to the latest figures published by the Office for National Statistics (2021a), life expectancy at birth in the UK in 2018–2020 was 79.0 years for males and 82.9 years for female, so creating a median point of life in the UK today would be 39.5 years for men, and 41.5 years for women. Other authors have considered midlife to be a bounded period of time rather than a specific age. Daniel Levinson studied middle-aged men in the US in the late 1960s and early 1970s, and he identified the midlife 'transition' as beginning at age 40 or 41 and lasting about five years (1978, p 191). He claimed that the midlife transition was unlikely to 'begin before age 38 or after 43' (1978, p 191). Across the literature, most situate the midlife period somewhere between 40 and 60 years old.

There has been a tendency for academic research to focus on the experiences at either end of the life course spectrum, with academic advancements in childhood studies and in gerontology. Benson (1997, p 2) suggests that this is perhaps because, unlike old age and childhood, midlife has no fixed start or end point and that it is those in midlife 'who provide the norms and values against which other groups seek to assert their separate identities'. It wasn't until the 1980s when Mike Featherstone and Mike Hepworth really started to take midlife seriously in the social sciences and brought this previously under-researched area of 'midlife' firmly into the academic consciousness. The one thing that is generally agreed upon by those who have made attempts to define midlife is that it signifies an important transition point in the life course. Midlife became synonymous with the term 'midlife crisis' following Jaques's coining of the phrase in his 1965 paper 'Death and the Midlife Crisis', yet generally the definition of the term 'midlife crisis' is still relatively unclear and has been commonly defined through popular myths and cultural stereotypes.

In my previous research into the midlife period, 'The Negotiation of Midlife' (Morgan Brett, 2011), I found that one of the defining features of midlife was an increased personal mortality awareness and existential thought, triggered by the shift in generational positioning. A generational shift involves the increasing agedness and eventual loss of the generation above and changes in the lives of the generation below. Life events such as the death of parents and other older relatives as well as children reaching adulthood and leaving the family home are commonly experienced in midlife. Elliot Jaques (1965) considered these changes to be a fundamental element of the midlife period, claiming that

> A new set of external circumstances has to be met. The first phase of adult life has been lived. Family and occupation have become established (or ought to have become established unless the individual's adjustments has gone seriously awry); parents have grown old, and children are at the thresholds of adulthood. Youth and childhood are past and gone, and demand to be mourned. (p 506)

What is interesting in this quotation is what Jaques termed 'a new set of external circumstances', which, for him, included the witnessing of ageing parents and the associated changing family roles, responsibilities, and dynamics. I began to realise that witnessing age-related changes in a parent can trigger age-awareness and can create general anxieties about health and physical appearance amongst adult children, whilst also revealing a deeper level of existential anxiety and concerns about ageing and the future.

The generational shift

One of the major challenges faced during the midlife phase of the life course is the generational shift and, consequently, facing Jaques's (1965) 'new set of external circumstances'. The generational shift sees the upward movement of the generations, which, for those in midlife, places them higher up in the hierarchy of the family tree (Sprang and McNeil, 1995), and this can impact on the way in which family roles and relationships are arbitrated. A shift to the oldest generational position in the family when parents die can evoke a range of emotions, from increased sense of responsibility, maturity, and wisdom to feelings of vulnerability, insecurity, and anxiety. It can also have an effect on the way people think about their own ageing process and mortality. When the older generation dies and the midlife individual moves into the older position, there may be the sense that they are next in line and the generational buffer between them and death has now gone. Taylor and Norris (1995, p 31) write that 'The loss of the role of son or daughter pushes middle-aged adults into the realisation that they are now the oldest generation, the next in line to die'. Marshall (2004, p 352) writes that, 'The consequences of the death of a parent are wide-ranging for the individual, perhaps prompting the adult children to examine their lives more closely, reassessing priorities and considering their own mortality as they move to the eldest generation in the family.'

Many sociological and psychological theorists across the decades have recognised the significant impact that a parent's death can have on someone in midlife, particularly regarding the feelings of vulnerability that result from increased mortality awareness. Spillius (1988, p 234), for example, suggested that until this point the individual has unconsciously believed in their immortality, but at this point death becomes 'a more realistic possibility'. Umberson (2003, p 131) writes that 'the death of a parent highlights the reality of our own individual mortality, especially since it is most likely to occur in middle adulthood, when our concerns about death are already on the rise', and notes that 'the adult child joins the next generation in line for death' (Umberson, 2003, p 50). Sprang and McNeil note that 'such a death brings to the fore one's own mortality … when a parent dies the adult child is next in line, the buffer is gone' (1995, p 21).

There are cultural conceptions about the normative transitions in the life course and when particular life events should take place, one of which is that death is expected in a natural order. When the older generation die first there is a sense of timeliness about their deaths; things are at least occurring in the 'right' order, even if this means that the midlife generation is now the next in line. This idea of the 'timeliness' of older parents' deaths is something which is explored in more detail in Chapter 6, 'The loss of parents in later life'. D'Epinay et al (2010, p 303) write that 'death is expected to respect the generational order'. Adult children in my research projects were aware of a shift in the generational structure of their family when their parents died. But for those who had one or more healthy parent, there was more reason to deny thoughts about their own deaths and to postpone thinking about ageing and death. There was an expectation that death would occur in the natural order, with the oldest in the family tree dying first; consequently, the healthy parents represented a psychological buffer between them and death. With the expectation that death would occur in the natural order with the oldest in the family tree dying first, respondents with healthy parents felt that they had little to worry about. Adult child Anna (aged 46) was a particular interesting example of this. Both of her parents were alive and in relatively good health. Her parents were divorced and lived separately, neither requiring any care assistance from her. Her dad, aged 70, lived in sheltered accommodation and still worked full time. Her mother became a nun and lived in a convent in relatively good health. Unusually, Anna also had a grandmother who was still alive. Her generational buffer was relatively robust in comparison to many other people interviewed. For Anna it seemed unnecessary to give any thought to her own death because, with a generation above her, if nature acted as expected, they would die before her. This safety net served to protect her from existential anxiety. She said:

> 'I mean in some ways, with my parents still, I think, well, my parents are still here, so for us to be discussing death and things for our own deaths seems a bit, I don't know, not stupid but irrelevant because my parents are still here. We haven't taken the mantle up, so to speak, to become the older generation yet, that is the only way I can put it. There is a line to follow.'

Umberson (2003) writes that 'the death of a parent is about the end of one generation and the passing of a torch to the next generation' (Umberson, 2003, p 131), and Petersen and Rafuls (1998, p 501) write that 'an adult child often must transition to becoming the standard bearer for the family as the "oldest" generation in the family, and with the assumption of this new generational role comes additional responsibilities to family members that might previously have accrued to the parental generation'. This is something which Anna was aware of but not yet ready to do whilst her parents were alive. This natural order is re-enforced by her grandmother's presence, "I have got a grandmother. So, you see, I am third in line! [Laughs] Back of the queue! Do you know what I mean?" Being at the 'back of the generation queue' for Anna gave her a psychological advantage, according to Marks et al (2007, p 1614) who wrote that 'those who have two primary affectional/attachment bond figures alive in their lives, might be expected to have a well-being advantage in adulthood that has been previously underestimated'.

However, even the witnessing of one's parents ageing process can thrust midlife adults into realising that they may soon become part of the older generation. Although both of 49-year-old Angela's parents were alive, witnessing age-related changes in her parents had begun to create anxieties about her own ageing process. Angela recalled:

> 'I saw my dad last week for this day out, for the first time I, the way he was walking and the way he was looking, he's lost a lot of weight you see, and I thought "My God dad, you look old!" and that's the first time I've really taken stock of how he was walking and how he was looking and that frightened me because I'm thinking, especially because of the way my thoughts are, I thought "Oh my God!" because I see everything happening in stages and everything and I think everything and everybody moves on a stage to another level don't they? And I thought "Oh my God, my dad's moved on to that next level!", which means I now shunt up and take his place! And that frightens me!'

Angela had become intensely aware of 'shunting' up the generations and appeared fearful of what that implied. Although her parents had not died, it was the recognition that they had aged which triggered Angela's mortality awareness and existential anxiety. She also later said, "I suppose they've always been immortal, which is silly because they're ageing in front of me". This statement was like an infantile phantasy about the indestructibility of her loved object; a phantasy of immortality for those she loves and immortality for herself. However, the reality of her parent's ageing and, in parallel, her own ageing has now begun to disrupt her phantasy, and this frightens her. This was reflective of her fears for her parent's mortality as well as her own and the feelings of loss and bereavement that these changes are inevitably going to bring. Parents may be taken for granted in everyday life and it can be frightening to realise that this relationship will not continue indefinitely and may soon come to an end.

Existential anxiety

Existential anxiety refers to a preoccupation about the meanings, choices, and directions one's life might take. This form of anxiety is particularly heightened during the midlife period when questions arise about the purposefulness of life so far and fears about the future and death are also brought to the fore. Anxiety is rooted in a fundamental fear of death; Arthur (2004, p 70) writes 'the psychoanalytic school and many of its philosophic successors agree that death is the basic source of all anxiety, the terror that haunts all human activity'.

Elliot Jaques (1965) first established a link between a fear of death and the midlife crisis and argued that the midlife crisis is advanced by the increasing awareness of the inevitability of one's own death. In this phase of the life course, the psychological self-deception of immortality begins to weaken and there is an increase in time awareness and a realisation that death is a more realistic possibility. He writes, 'the reality and inevitability of one's own eventual personal death, that is the central and crucial feature of the midlife phase' (1965, p 506). Furthermore, he pessimistically writes, 'the paradox is that of entering the prime of life, the stage of fulfilment, but at the same time the prime and fulfilment are dated. Death lies beyond' (Jaques, 1965, p 506). Literature across many different academic disciplines has recognised an increase in mortality awareness during the midlife period. The psychologist Daniel Levinson noted an increase in death awareness in midlife. He said:

> [A]t 40 a man knows more deeply than ever that he is going to die … His death is not simply an abstract, hypothetical event. An unpredictable accident or illness could take his life tomorrow. Even another thirty

years does not seem so long: more years now lie behind than ahead. (1978, p 215)

The historian Peter Laslett also wrote about a 'sense of a collective future' which is 'held by those whose personal future is inevitably short' (1996, pp x–xi). Psychoanalyst Pearl King addressed some of the 'pressures which seem to operate as sources of anxiety and concern during the second half of the life cycle', which included 'the inevitability of their own death and the realization that they may not now be able to achieve the goals they set for themselves, and that what they can achieve and enjoy in life may be limited, with consequent feelings of depression or deprivation' (King, 1980, p 154). The psychoanalyst Carl Jung (1930, p 397) described midlife as the peak of the sun's crescent, with only a descent into sunset beyond – 'at the stroke of noon the descent begins'. And, finally, the sociologist and thanotologist Michael C. Kearl argued that midlife represents a period in which the individual starts to realise the inevitability of their own death and for some people this means that the countdown to death has begun (1989, p 465).

But why is mortality awareness such a significant feature of midlife? Certainly, much has been written about the denial of death throughout the life course. Freud wrote about how people tend to 'shelve death' (1917) and avoid thinking about it. Arthur writes, 'an established corpus of scholarly research shows how terror of death is so overwhelming, to our conscious selves, that we repress it' (Arthur, 2004, p 68). Cultural anthropologist Ernest Becker in his seminal 1973 text *The Denial of Death*, argued that human beings have a unique insight into their fate; that they know with certainty that they will one day die. This generates an enormous responsibility to preserve life and a conscious knowledge of this responsibility can lead to great anxiety. Becker claimed that this knowledge is so unbearable that virtually all of our daily activity is an attempt to deny and overcome our fate. He claimed that the individual 'literally drives himself into a blind obliviousness with social games, psychological tricks, and personal preoccupations' (1973, p 27). Despite the anxiety death provokes, Becker pointed out that to fear death constantly would hinder the effective functioning of human life, so for the most part of their lives people keep busy in their daily routines: they think about other things, they ignore death, they deny death, they leave thinking about death until another day and they think of death as something which always happens to someone else. Arthur (2004, p 73) expands this: 'Becker is right; that one of the meaner aspects of our natural human narcissism is that we feel that practically everyone is expendable, except us.'

In the mid section of the life course death becomes harder to deny as the psychological self-deception that Becker (1973) referred to begins to weaken and those in midlife begin to realise that time is passing by more quickly and death is becoming a more realistic possibility. I propose that a fear of death in midlife is increased not simply because of the number of years that have passed and, through counting, how many are left, because this would simply mean that we became increasingly fearful the older we become, but rather a fear of death becomes particularly intensified during this midlife period and that it lessens or is experienced in a newly transformed way beyond midlife and into old age. And one of the reasons for this is that midlife is experienced as a series of 'losses'. Jaques (1965) acknowledged that change and loss, related to the generational shift in particular, can contribute to an increased fear of death in midlife. He wrote that 'the sense of the agedness of parents, coupled with the maturing of children into adults, contributes strongly to the sense of ageing – the sense that it is one's own turn next to grow old and die' (1965, pp 506, 510). Becker (1973) argued that a denial of death is a psychological defence mechanism used to protect against an existential threat and that the individual employs techniques to avoid thinking about death. Yet it is the loss or death of a parent which can finally breach these defences, confront the adult child with their own personal mortality, and refine their perceptions of who they are and what they want from life.

I am aware that these arguments portray a rather depressing and pessimistic view of midlife, so can we claim that all those in midlife are so aware and as afraid of death as these theorists would lead us to believe? Moreover, is having increased mortality awareness and existential thought always a negative psychological state to be in? Certainly, midlife is a critical transition period in which loss is a prominent feature; however, it is possible for this to also become a period of growth and self-actualisation. It has been argued that the fear of death is a prime motivator for human activity. Becker stated that 'of all things that move man, one of the principal ones is his terror of death' (1973, p 11). Viorst asserted that 'the emotional knowledge that we surely will die someday can heighten and fine-tune our sense of the present moment' (1986, p 306). When emotional knowledge is broadened in midlife, through physical and mental changes, this can lead to an increased sense of the present moment and an acknowledgment that one should make the most of it. Calhoun et al (2010, p 128) suggest that:

> When a death occurs, people can report that there is a realisation that the end of life may be sooner than they think, or that they must make the most of what time they have. This appreciation of life, living it more vividly, may be difficult for some people to sustain, but it is sometimes consolidated into new habits of living more deliberately rather than routinely.

There is often a tension between this existential anxiety and fear of death, and the potential for growth and self-actualisation, which links into Erikson's (1963) seventh life stage with the ego tasks of 'generativity vs stagnation'.

Generativity involves paying back society for the things it has given to you through working hard and raising a family. It encompasses 'procreativity, productivity and creativity' and is about 'guiding the next generation or whatever in a given case may become the absorbing object of a parental kind of responsibility'. This may include creative pursuits, the generation of new ideas, and personal identity development (Erikson, 1963, p 231). Interestingly, Jaques (1965) also noted increased creativity in many people during midlife. He studied 310 artistic geniuses and he found that although the process of creativity is more laboured it was often the time when the greatest works of art were produced. Midlife requires a degree of urgency for some aspect of generative achievement or else it risks entering into an existence of self-absorption and isolation. This is generativity's opposing ego-quality which Erikson termed 'stagnation'.

The drive towards generativity can mean that the adult child is in a phase of life where they desire change and want to create a legacy which lives beyond them, giving their life meaning and purpose. This may mean a return to education, guiding younger generations, changing career or seeking promotion, travelling, or transforming into a more authentic version of one's own self-identity. But generativity can also be a form of 'care' and giving something back through the act of caregiving. Yet, simultaneously, becoming a carer for an older parent is psychologically confronting. Increasing mortality awareness, changes in role identity, and fluctuations in roles and responsibilities can mean that the adult child can lose a sense of who they are, and 'stagnated' as to what direction they should take. Here lies Erikson's psychosocial conflict.

The term 'ontological security', first introduced by R.D. Laing (1961) and later used by Giddens (2001 [1991]), refers to the repetition of taken-for-granted practices which give people a sense of order and continuity in relation to everyday events. The psychological mechanism of ontological security plays a fundamental role in creating what Giddens termed a 'protective cocoon' (2001 [1991]) from existential anxieties threatening the individual's integrity of self and the effective functioning of society in general. 'Ontological security "brackets out" potential occurrences which, were the individual seriously to contemplate them, would produce a paralysis of the will, or feelings of engulfment' (2001 [1991], p 3). If an individual has a strong sense of ontological security they can proceed in their lives with a sense of safety and security about their lives and the world around them. Ontological security can be disrupted by contingencies, moments of realisation, and untimely deaths.

This concept of ontological security is important to consider when thinking about caring for an older parent, because a parent's sudden health crisis, a drastic change in life circumstances, a sudden shift in role or responsibility, or the unexpected death of a parent can all shake the adult child to the core, impacting significantly on their mental well-being and behaviours. For instance, if a parent dies suddenly or prematurely, this can shock the adult child into new health behaviours in order to prevent the same thing happening to them. Umberson (2003, p 98) wrote that 'recognition of personal mortality may lead to very practical behaviours in terms of preparing for one's own death'. Respondents in the research for this book demonstrated this through behaviours such as the urgent preparation of wills, having discussions with family about death, and considering future funeral plans. Sharon (aged 54) was one particular participant who had become profoundly aware of her own mortality as a result of her own father's premature death and her mum's advanced ageing. She told me:

> 'Because my father died when he was 55, I've never really thought I'd have a long life. I know that sounds very morbid, but I just never have. And now I'm getting older, and I want to get fitter. I see the way my mum is, and obviously I know you can't prevent that happening, but, you know, any kind of old age ailments and things I'm just going to try and put off.'

I asked her, "Have you given much thought to your own death?" She replied, "Oh, all the time. Every day! Sometimes I don't expect to wake up. I was only 21 when my dad died, so it has been almost every day, but it's not in a morbid way, I guess you're just aware of death all the time." She went on to describe the impact this has had on her everyday behaviours. Sharon does not have children and has very little family around her, so for her it was especially important to have her affairs in order in case someone external had to deal with them. She went on to say, "Sometimes I think I must keep the flat tidy in case I die, and so other people are going to see it".

Sociological and psychological theorists have recognised the significant impact that a parent's death can have on someone in midlife, particularly regarding the feelings of vulnerability that result from increased mortality awareness. Spillius (1988, p 234), for example, suggested that until this point the individual has unconsciously believed in their immortality, but at this point death becomes 'a more realistic possibility'. And Umberson (2003, p 131) asserted that 'the death of a parent highlights the reality of our own individual mortality, especially since it is most likely to occur in middle adulthood, when our concerns about death are already on the rise'.

Chapter summary

Midlife is a period of the life course with distinct challenges. It can be a time for self-actualisation and growth, but it also a time of loss and grief when witnessing the ageing of parents. A sense of a generational shift brings forth an acute awareness of one's own death too, leading to urgency to accomplish life goals. This period of life is about coming to terms, not only with death and existential anxiety, but with loss and disappointment. Losses are faced sporadically throughout the life course, but it is the unique state of culminating losses which is a feature of midlife. It is a time when parents are reaching advanced ages or dying, and the children's generation are growing up and moving on. There may be a reduction in physical capabilities, and recognition to the limitations of achievement, and personal goals have to be acknowledged or redirected (Morgan Brett, 2011). The losses which arise from this period of change and instability often reawaken old threats, anxieties, and defences which were first experienced in the early infantile stages. Feelings of abandonment, threats to attachment juxtaposed by the need for independence and autonomy, are the original dilemmas of infancy but are replayed in midlife. Midlife is about the resolution of this conflict, as was once necessary in infancy, but it is now with a new insight into and understanding of death.

In the next chapter we will explore the experience of informal caregiving for an older parent, and the implications this new role has on the adult child's sense of identity. We will also look at sibling dynamics and the coordination and division of care labour and how this can reignite historical, infantile dynamics within family systems.

2

Becoming a carer

With an ageing population in the UK, family members are increasingly finding themselves in the positions of informal caregiving. These caregiving roles evolve over time and change with the increasing agedness and associated frailty of the older relative, until the point comes when decisions have to be made about transitioning an older person into a care home where they can receive more intense or specialised support.

This chapter begins the journey of the adult child becoming a 'carer', and the initial stages of transitioning a parent into care. The first challenge involves an identity shift for the adult child from 'son or daughter' to becoming a 'carer' and how this feels like a role reversal – becoming a parent's parent – with important consequences for their relationship with their parent. Family dynamics can change too when the labour of care is divided between sibling pairings or groups, reigniting historical rivalries or alliances which were previously played out in childhood between brothers and sisters.

We begin the chapter by exploring what it means to 'care', the very definition of which has been subject of significant debate. Care involves a range of instrumental tasks, but it also involves significant emotional labour, and this emotional work in particular has traditionally been considered a female occupation – a daughter's domain – when caring for an older parent. Feminist scholars have redefined care to better recognise the emotional work and relational experience involved in the care relationship and have advocated for a more egalitarian distribution of care, not just within families, but by society as a whole.

Care and gendered expectations

Fine and Glendinning (2005, p 617) write that care 'is a social concept that defies rigid definition, yet is helpful as both a normative, aspirational guide and a term for describing our behaviour', considering care to be a set of practices which we carry out to provide assistance to the health and welfare of another. These practices may include physical activities of care, social transactions of care between people, and mental states of caring for another (Fine and Glendinning, 2005). The Care Collective define care as 'a social capacity and activity involving the nurturing of all that is necessary for the welfare and flourishing of life' (The Care Collective, 2020, p 5). Willyard et al (2008, p 1674) suggest that caregiving involves a broad spectrum of activities under two primary categories, 'activities of daily living' and 'instrumental activities of daily living'. Activities of daily living might include providing personal care, bathing, dressing, feeding, supervising medication, and companionship. Instrumental activities of daily living can include tasks such as taking care of financial decisions and paying bills, and household activities such as cleaning, cooking, shopping, and coordinating medical care. Adult children involved in these tasks are considered 'primary carers' (Willyard et al, 2008, p 1674). When caring for ageing parents these caregiving activities may start small – a brief visit, taking a parent out, or preparing a meal – but with a parent's advancing age, a caregiving role can intensify and impact more significantly upon the adult child's daily life. This range of care definitions highlights both a variety of activities and tasks but also a range of interactions and socio-emotional forms of support. As we will come to see in this chapter, the ways in which care roles are defined and valued in family systems and within society is dependent upon underlying biased expectations around gender and women's roles.

The term 'carer' came into public consciousness in the early 1960s, through a concern about the under-appreciation of women's unpaid care work within the family. There has been a long-held assumption that women are naturally 'caring', that care work is 'women's work', and traditionally women have been expected to adopt a 'caring role' within the traditional family establishment (The Care Collective, 2020). In 1963 Reverend Mary Webster highlighted the plight of informal carers (primarily women) who were challenged by formal working whilst also carrying out the unpaid labour of caring for older parents. In 1965, Reverend Webster established the National Council for the Single Woman and Her Dependents (NCSWD), which later became Carers UK, but it was not until the Carer's Act 2004 that the specific needs of carers beyond their caring responsibilities was recognised (Carers UK, 2022).

Tronto (1993) distinguished four phases of the caregiving role and Sevenhuijsen (2003) mapped the corresponding moral values to each care phase (they are italicised here for ease of explanation). First Tronto (1993) wrote that 'caring about' is about recognising a need for care with the related moral value of *attentiveness*. The second phase is 'caring for', which involves taking *responsibility* that the care need is met. This involves being able to respond on an emotional level to someone's need for care. Tronto's next care phase is 'care giving', which refers to a *competency* in identifying and carrying out the practical tasks required to meet the caring needs. It is worth noting that Lloyd (2012, p 39) suggests that *competence* in this context does not mean simply that those who are in the caring role are educated and trained to care, but that it refers to the provision of resources in order to ensure that carers can carrying out their role to a high standard. The fourth dimension of care is 'care receiving', which refers to an interaction between the caregiver and care receiver and an evaluation of the *responsiveness* to the care need. Later, in 2013, Tronto made the addition of 'caring with', which refers to ongoing cycle of care upon which trust has been built. In this phase the individual begins to realise – and *trust* – that they can rely upon others to participate in their care activities with *integrity*. Sevenhuijsen (2003, p 184) writes that 'these four values: *attentiveness*, *responsibility*, *competence* and *responsiveness* form the core of the ethic of care as moral orientation and thus of care as social practice' (italics my own) and along with *trust* and *integrity* they form a framework for an ethics of care.

Feminist literature has focused on the disproportionate amount of care that women carry out (Gilligan, 1982; Tronto, 1993; Sevenhuijsen, 2003). Informal family carers are more likely to be female (60 per cent) (Foley, 2022, p 8). And even in the labour market, the majority of paid caregivers are women. Around 80 per cent of all jobs in adult social care are carried out by women; the proportion in direct care and support-providing jobs is higher, at 85–95 per cent (The Kings Fund, 2022). Caring is seen as a woman's occupation. Typically, women tend to take responsibility for more intensive and time-consuming forms of care, including personal care, meal preparation, laundry, and other household activities, while men are more likely to assist with financial matters, heavy chores, and transportation needs (Chappell and Penning, 2005). Women (daughters/sisters in the family group) are more likely to maintain and facilitate family relations, and women are more likely to take on intensive caregiving roles for their ageing parents.

Yet, care roles for women today typically have to be performed alongside paid labour. Since the 1950s, in industrialised countries women have increasingly entered the workforce, yet even today there is an inequality within the labour market. Women face structural disadvantages such as economic vulnerability, increased expectations to manage childcare, and lower incomes for comparative roles in the workplace. Women are frequently expected to adjust their work schedules to adapt to the care demands of children and or older relatives, 'yet, they are disproportionately employed in occupations that offer limited flexibility with respect to such arrangements' (Chappell and Penning, 2005, p 459). There is also often an expectation that women (usually daughters caring for ageing parents) will take leave from the workplace to take up care roles, but then find it more difficult to re-enter the job market when their caring responsibilities have come to an end (Westwood and Daly, 2016, p 27).

Feminist research since the early 1980s has problematised the definition of care, challenging this normative expectation that women should shoulder the burden of care. Feminist scholars have sought to highlight the need to make visible the huge amount of unpaid care that women bear within their homes and families. They have redefined care, placing greater value on the emotional and relational dimensions of caring as opposed to the more instrumental, task-driven characterisation that care has previously held.

The emotional labour of care

As we have seen, care defies easy definition and is often thought of, and treated as, a task-based activity, sometimes at the neglect of the emotional aspect of the care relationship. Yet, caring for a parent in later life can elicit complex emotional responses which include empathy, love and affection, as well as feelings of disgust, revulsion, shame, and fear. Acknowledgement of, and the ability to work through, these feelings is a crucial part of the caregiving relationship, and if they are not properly dealt with, defensive care practices can arise (Menzies Lyth, 1960).

Feminist perspectives, such as that of Gilligan (1982) and Sevenhuijsen (2003) place emotional labour at the heart of care. Sevenhuijsen (2003, p 186) writes that 'the ability and willingness to place oneself in the perceptions and viewpoints of others is indispensable in practising care and responsibility'. However, the emotional elements of care such as empathy, relationality, and affection are harder to quantify, measure, and value in a system of statistics, outcomes, and measurements. Land and Himmelweit (2010, p 17) write that:

> Care is a quintessentially 'soft' product whose essential characteristics are not easily measured. It is possible to monitor the attainment of certain physical tasks, such as, whether a client has been bathed or taken their medicine. Market-driven provision, in its drive for efficiency, will tend to meet these measurable outputs and economise on the less tangible aspects of good care. But these are of the very essence of good care, which in nearly all cases needs to include the development of a warm relationship between care provider and recipient. Such things are hard to monitor and necessarily tend to fall by the wayside in the pursuit of market-led 'efficiency'. (Gilbert, 2002; Stone, 2000)

Carol Gilligan (1982) first recognised this devaluation of emotional skills held by women in caregiving roles. In her book *In a Different Voice*, she challenged Kohlberg's (1971) study of moral reasoning which found that females obtained a lower 'moral judgement rating' than males, thus marking females at a lower stage of moral development than males. However, Gilligan (1982) found that when both males and females in her study were asked to reason through examples of moral dilemmas, the female participants spoke to her in a 'different voice', favouring the language of connection, relationships, care, and sensitivity, which contrasted to the male language of rule-based justice, regulations, and a morality of rights. Instead of considering dominant philosophical traditions of ethics as a set of abstract, universal principles based upon competency, moral principles of 'right and wrong' and obligations, Gilligan (1987) proposed that the feminist ethics of care should focus on the ways in which ethics are understood on a contextual level and that they should relate to the circumstances and moral dilemmas faced by people in their everyday lives. Translating this into a discussion about the care of older parents means that we should encourage contextually responsive and relational forms of care which are adaptable and based in love, goodwill (a form of care favoured and valued by women, or daughters in this context), in addition to, or in place of, care practices bound by rules, power-based structures, and ideals (favoured by males, or sons in this context). It is this privileging of relational care which is central to feminist ethics.

The framework for a feminist ethics of care emphasises interdependency, relationality, and interconnectivity (Sevenhuijsen, 2003). Care does not have to be, nor arguably should be, something that is done unto another, as this places the care receiver and caregiver in unequal positions of power and control. Sevenhuijsen (1997) highlighted that in Western society there has been a growing preoccupation on the virtues of autonomy, independence, and individualisation, which means that to be 'dependent' upon another is to be seen as a point of failure. However, being dependent with the need to be cared for by another is part of the human condition. Dependency and interdependency is something which is inherent across the whole of the life course (Tronto, 1993; Lloyd, 2012). Molyneaux et al (2011, p 422) critiqued the term carer, suggesting that it implies a sense of burden and devalues and ignores the experience of the individual who is cared for and 'polarises two individuals who would otherwise work together'. Rather, a feminist ethics of care perspective suggests that care should be 'best understood as something which is the product or outcome of a relationship' (Fine and Glendinning, 2005, p 616). Gilligan (1984, p 73) wrote about a 'web of connection', which is about an interconnectivity of relationships and taking care of one another. Kittay (1999, pp 67–8) developed the concept of 'nested-dependencies' which involve 'exchange-based reciprocity' and take into account both the needs of the caregiver and those of the care receiver.

These interdependencies sit within broader societal structure in which the care relationship is reliant upon society for the provision of resources and support. The Care Collective (2020, p 6) states that care cannot be effectively carried out unless both the caregiver and the care receiver are supported, and this cannot happen unless care is 'cultivated, shared and resourced on an egalitarian basis' and is 'neither exploited nor devalued'. Sevenhuijsen (2003, p 193) promotes the term 'caring citizenship', which reflects an ideal in which 'caring is part of collective agency in the public sphere'. A feminist ethics of care argues that it is essential to incorporate care into the definition of active social citizenship. For example, The Care Collective (2020, p 44) uses the term 'promiscuous care', which refers to caring openly and freely, whilst also building in systems and institutional arrangements which are 'capacious and agile enough to recognise and resource wider forms of care at the level of kinship'. One such system that I refer to in this book is the work of My Home Life England and in particular the related national initiative Care Home Friends and Neighbours (CHFaNs) that encourages connections between care homes and their local communities in order that the whole community plays a role in caring for those who live and work in the home, ensuring that they have the best possible quality of life (My Home Life England, 2022).

Sibling coordination of caregiving

Gendered division of care was evident amongst the adult children within their sibling groups in the research undertaken for this book. Shmotkin (1999, p 474) writes that 'following very early modes of identification and socialization (Chodorow, 1978), women tend to assume the role of "kin-keepers" who maintain and facilitate family relations (Hagestad, 1986; Troll and Bengtson, 1982)'. With parental care duties to be fulfilled, there can be some uncertainty about who should undertake what roles and responsibilities within a family system. Some cooperative sibling groups demonstrated coordination and a clear division of labour, the dynamics of the group strengthening when having to pull together to fulfil the caregiving tasks for an ageing parent. Yet, other sibling groups exhibited a complete breakdown of relationships when caring for an ageing parent, as historic sibling tensions, which perhaps had been put aside or ignored as they had grown older, were reignited and revisited when they were forced together to make difficult decisions (Khodyakov and Carr, 2009).

In my research, brothers tended to take on more instrumental roles such as a taking charge of financial affairs, and it was the sisters who took on the more personal, intimate, or emotional care roles. Sisters were expected to be more involved with the activities of daily living than their brothers, as these tasks were deemed as being within the domain of a woman's expertise. Lily (aged 57) recognised this in her sibling group, cynically saying, "I do think that women get dumped upon." However, she described a relatively well-functioning family 'team' and a clear division of labour amongst her sibling group when caring for their 87-year-old mother who was living with dementia. She said, "We had to come together on this, we felt we had to," and continued, "we had our roles, and I think, you know, I mean, there's an awful lot of politics under the surface which can erupt at any minute, but I think with this – and also when my father died – we were all absolutely a team." She went on to describe how her sibling group had distributed the caregiving roles:

'My brother is an actuary, so he took care of the finances, which is great, because I didn't want to do that. My older sister did the sort of visiting, which I didn't want to do either. And I did the organising, which nobody else wanted to do. And my younger sister actually knew what the hell was going on, and she was very, that was good. But she was in America, so that was very, very difficult for her, for us, for everybody.'

Jilly (aged 68) described a similar arrangement with her brother when caring for their now 99-year-old mother. She said:

'My brother does all the financial side, so he often talks to her, or asks her to keep her bank statements. He deals with the solicitor, or whatever, accountant thing. So, he does that side, and I do the more personal side. Certainly, at Christmas I do all the cards that she should send to people, and birthdays, we keep up with people – all the family, cousins and people, her nephews, and nieces – and I do all that with her, and for her. So that's important.'

Sibling groups with a strong sense of their existing family roles, pre-existing expectations, and a strong sense of what each member's individual skills were better able to define the care roles within the family system. The birth order of siblings was another important factor in how responsibility was delegated in families (Petersen and Rafuls, 1998, p 499). This was evident in Fred's sibling dyad. Fred (aged 56) had a good relationship with his older brother, who was seven years older, and had been happy to let his brother do all of the care and arrangements for their parents before they died when they were in their mid 80s. It did not seem to have had any significant impact on their sibling relationship according to Fred, but it did seem that Fred had fallen back into an almost child-like relationship again with his brother, where his big brother would take charge of the difficult situations and Fred would stay quietly in the background as the 'little brother'.

Sibling groups, although somewhat transformed over their adulthood years, were likely to have the same undercurrent of early sibling dynamics when faced with a family crisis such as caring for an ageing parent. There were unresolved difficult feelings of parental favouritism, ambivalence, rivalry, power struggles, and competitiveness, and these were re-enacted through regressive acts and phantasies. Jilly (aged 68) recognised this in her relationship with her brother, saying: "We have a slightly strained relationship, but that isn't anything, nothing to do with my mother, though. No. It's just, we haven't really bonded since childhood somehow."

Where there were inequalities in the division of care labour amongst sibling groups, non- or lesser-participating siblings were sometimes asked to contribute more to the role or were excluded from the family boundaries. The distribution of care tasks are rarely equal, but they need to be *considered* 'fair' within the group. The contextual factors of birth order, gender, employment status, geographical proximity, and childcare duties were all considered when making the decisions about what felt 'fair'. Personality types were also a way to excuse a lack of contribution or justify a contributory role. However, if contributions were not perceived as fair, this led to anger, conflict, frustration, resentment, and resignation towards those less-involved siblings. Further, those siblings who contribute less may feel guilt and shame, or even frustrated and left out of/pushed out of decision-making processes and underappreciated for the contributions that they do make. From a study which looked at the inequity in parent care among siblings, Ingersoll-Dayton et al (2003) recognised that there can be a 'double jeopardy', with feelings of anger at the inequity and feelings of guilt about the negative emotions felt towards a sibling. They write, 'One possible explanation is that when primary-caregiver siblings get angry with their less involved siblings, they feel guilty because their negative emotions are inconsistent with the solidarity that they expect to feel with their siblings (Lerner et al, 1991)' (Ingersoll-Dayton et al, 2003, p 206).

Sharon (aged 54) and her sister Lucy (aged 57) had had a relatively dysfunctional sister relationship since childhood, which was exacerbated by the care decisions that needed to be made for their mother (aged 83) when she developed dementia. Twenty years previous, Lucy had moved 250 miles away from the area where her mum and sister lived following a family argument. As their mother aged and her physical and mental health declined, she required increasing levels of care in her own home. Sharon worked full time and found the care burden too great to manage on her own. Sharon had been granted lasting power of attorney and made the decision for her mum to move into a local care home. However, her sister Lucy disagreed with the decision, despite not taking on any of the care responsibilities. Sharon said, "My big thing was always that my sister was really, just not helping at all, and hindering instead." When their mother's house had to be cleared of possessions the resentment between them grew. Sharon recalled:

'I tried to maintain a bit of a relationship with her, but the biggest thing I think was trying to clear out the house by myself. She had been in that house for 50 years, and my mother never threw anything away, ever! So that was a big job to do by yourself, and she didn't want to help me, so I just kind of, I sort of gradually, I didn't have any arguments with her, I just gradually stopped contacting her really, and she stopped contacting me.'

She goes on to say:

'She didn't want me to sell the house, she didn't want my mum to go in the Home, but she wasn't here, she didn't want to help. I did say to her, "Why don't you take her to live in your house? You've got a big four-bedroom house, you know, your kids have left, why, you know, why can't you?" But she didn't want that!'

Ingersoll-Dayton et al (2003, p 209) observed in their study that siblings who were providing more care for their parents 'tried to minimize their siblings' under-involvement by observing that they were psychologically incapable of providing care'. With Sharon this too seemed to be the case, with her describing Lucy as "not very well in the head", thus accounting for her lack of contribution, and expressing a desire to be left to her own decision-making with regards to their mum's care. Willyard et al (2008, p 1684) point out that 'if the caregiver develops a narrative that she is more endowed with these skills than her sibling(s), it only makes sense that she takes on the lion's share of the caregiving role'.

'Only children' seemed to have some advantage in caregiving. Without the often-conflicting input of other siblings, only children were able to take charge, feel more confident in their decision-making, have more autonomy about care choices, and more say on what happened to property and possessions. Only children reported increased bonds with parents, but also sometimes felt a little lonely in their situations due to a lack of social and emotional support. Coleen (aged 45), for example, would have liked a wider network of support but also recognised the benefits of lone caring for her 74-year-old father who had dementia. She said: "I did wish I had a husband/partner, whatever, just someone, just, not to take it all on, or brothers and sisters, although I do know from other friends who have been in this experience, that brothers and sisters don't always help, and sometimes they hinder."

Similarly, Hazel recognised the advantages of her singleton status: "It doesn't matter about siblings. There was only me making the decisions, not the only person visiting, but certainly the only person making the decisions and making everything happen." For Hazel, it was her wider network of support that was important. She had friends and neighbours who would pop by to see her mum in the care home, but ultimately the decision-making was Hazel's alone.

Dividing the care responsibilities for an ageing parent involves multi-layered family involvement and interconnections. Divisiveness amongst sibling groups and pairs can reignite childhood tensions and open old wounds, which can irreparably damage the relationship. However, it is important to take account of and to understand the positionality of each sibling and their individual circumstances. When well coordinated, each sibling can bring their own unique strength and skillset to the parent-care contribution. Although caring for a parent can be incredibly stressful and result in a caregiver burden, it can also be a deeply rewarding and positive experience.

Reciprocity in intergenerational care

Evidence from the literature along with evidence from my own research data collection suggest that a dominant theme in caring for an older parent is reciprocity, and the sense that an adult child feels a sense of duty, obligation, or 'paying back' for the care they received as a child from their parents (Wenzel and Poynter, 2014; Gans et al, 2009; Silverstein et al, 2006; Willyard et al, 2008). Wenzel and Poynter (2014, p 155) write that 'many parents simultaneously validated the cultural idea that children are obligated to take care of their parents and the belief that ageing parents should maintain their independence'. Gans et al (2009, p 634) found evidence in their research of the literature in this area that 'earlier parental investments in their young children are later reciprocated by instrumental assistance, suggesting a quid-pro-quo over the family life course' and 'by providing transfers earlier in life, parents build a sense of obligation in their children to reciprocate later in life'. However, for parents it can be difficult to accept that they may have to depend upon their own children in a way that their own parents depended upon them in the past, and cherished feelings of autonomy and independence can feel threatened by an increasing dependence upon their children.

Adult children, in my research, indicated that their role as a caregiver was influenced by the generations of care that came before them. Stark (1995) described this as a 'demonstration effect', which referred to upstream intergenerational transfers. The demonstration effect results in higher levels of instrumental and socio-emotional support provided to an older relative, when it is known that the older relative did that for their parents too. Sharon (aged 54) exemplifies this by saying, "My grandmother lived – my mum's mum – lived with us, so I've kind of, you know, gone down that generation." Alison (aged 63) was aware of care across her family generations. She remembered:

> 'It was a lovely thing to do, to be able to care for your mum like that. When you think that, you know she did this for me. She'd say, "You know, you don't have to do this for me. I'm old, and I'm not worth it" and "I ought to be doing things for you", but she obviously couldn't. We used to say, "Well, you did this for Granny and for Granddad and for Nanna", and "You did it for us when we were little".'

Alison was aware of the caregiving relationships that preceded hers with her mother and was perhaps demonstrating to the next generation (her own three children, in their 30s) what it meant to be a caregiver. Rob too described the care he provided for his mum as a form of 'payback'. He describes:

> 'I have to go and cut the grass for her and deadhead for her, things like this, I have to do her shopping for her. I take her out on Sundays, and

we go for a drive. It's all those things, but the amount of energy she put into me and also my family, it's a small payback really.'

Parental relationships are not always easy, and some adult children lived with parents who were unsupportive or, worse, abusive or neglectful in caring for their children. Lily, for example, struggled in particular with the intimate care aspects of supporting her mum, and she reflected upon this as almost a form of unconscious comeuppance for her mother's uncaring nature when Lily was a child. "I didn't want to be her nurturer, the parenting your parent sort of thing. I think there's probably something else going on, a sort of feeling of, 'You didn't nurture me so I'm not going to nurture you'." This shift of a parent adopting the child's role can be really difficult to cope with in these more dysfunctional relationships, and particularly when there is a societal and familial expectation that the adult child *should* care for their parent, regardless of the relationship.

Becoming a 'carer'

It can be physically and emotionally challenging to care for an older parent and adult children can find themselves thrust into a position of 'carer' without preparation or training and having to perform unfamiliar or undesirable tasks. Furthermore, this shift in caregiving activities can involve a change in personal identity. Piercy and Chapman (2001, p 391) write that 'identifying oneself as a caregiver to frail older adults requires some degree of role enactment'. The adult child has to become socialised to the role of a caregiver, and this has implications for how they view their relationship with their parent.

The term 'carer' is not always identified with by those giving, or even receiving care, suggesting that those being cared for may deny the presence of their 'carer' and consequently underestimate and under-appreciate the level of care that occurs in that relationship. One reason for this, Molyneaux et al (2011) suggest, is that the term 'carer' is complicated in that it is associated with a paid professional role and this goes beyond the role of the informal family carer. Barnes (2012, p 9) highlights the reluctance of some informal caregivers to identify themselves with the label of 'carer' in preference of 'emphasising instead their prior relationships' such as daughter or son. Sharon (aged 54), for example, described how she experienced this change in role title when caring for her ageing mother:

'I hated being called a "carer". Suddenly, I was a "carer". One day I was the daughter, and the next I was the carer, it was a real psychological blow. And I know there's nothing you can do about it, but suddenly you're given the responsibility. I found that quite difficult. I didn't like it at all. It's just like an official title that's bunged on you.'

Sharon was happy to take on a caring role for her mum and the responsibility that came with it, but the identity change from daughter to carer was unsettling.

Being labelled a 'carer' does not necessarily mean that this is a caring relationship. As noted in the previous section, in some circumstances the adult child may feel forced into an obligatory care relationship with someone that they do not emotionally care for. There may be an abusive history in the child–parent relationship and being thrust into that role can lead to additional conflict and stress. Wider family expectations around who *should* care for an older parent may be in conflict with how the adult child feels about that role. In addition, dementia can lead to personality changes and even aggressive behaviour which are uncharacteristic of the person with the condition, and adult children can find these changes in behaviour difficult to deal with too. Ruth's (aged 54) father has dementia and lives in a care home. She described this change: "It's just unpleasant sometimes. He can be verbally aggressive, but that's not with us. I've only experienced that once or twice, just a couple of times. He was never aggressive. He *was* a really gentle guy." Other adult children noticed (often frustrating) changes in personality as a consequence of dementia, and how this had affected the relationship they had with their parents. Jilly (aged 68) noticed that her relationship with her mum (aged 99) had changed: "Our relationship has only got worse because of her memory loss and her ageing. I can't have exactly the same kind of conversation I've had years ago, and it's completely understandable, but I do get sometimes quite depressed. I miss how she used to be." She went on to highlight this shifting dependency her mother had on her: "The relationship, it's deteriorated because she's dependent on me. Although she's here, she's dependent on what I say, and what I know, rather than herself." Annie (aged 70) also noticed this decline in the frustrating changes she experienced when communicating with her mum (aged 99). She said:

> 'It's hard because you feel that you're trying to explain things, but it's not going in. It's just the fact that there's no conversation really. You know, you just tell her one thing, and then something is said, and she says, "Well, you didn't tell me". I say, "I've just told, I've just told you!" You just have to repeat everything over and over again.'

If contact with an ageing parent is inconsistent, these personality changes can seem drastic, stark, and unnerving with every visit. And if there is a lack of awareness of the progression of a parent's decline, the blame for the changes is sometimes directed at the care home and its staff. This is discussed further in Chapter 5, 'Social connections and relationship building in residential care'.

Adult children often draw upon their existing parent–child structure to make sense of their new caregiver identity. Most frequently they noticed a shift in the relational dynamic between themselves and their parent, which played out as becoming a parent's parent. As a care home volunteer articulated, "It's like a role reversal. The children become the parents. It's tough for them, the families, really tough." This shift was also recognised by the older parents. Care home resident Coral (aged 84), for example, told me, "The balance has changed. Now, she's [her daughter] doing me the favours."

Patricia (aged 55) noticed that the roles have become reversed with her father. She says, "In later life when your roles reverse a bit … you are doing more for them than they are for you." Patricia had recognised a change in her father's character and sometimes found this changing role difficult to deal with. She described an incident when her father found out he was going blind: "I was holding him and cuddling him, and he was sobbing, and he was just frightened of going blind. And he says, 'What will I do, what will I do?'" She also described how her father had gone from being a strong character who would speak his mind to a quiet, meek man, and this had come as a shock to her. She invited him round for dinner a few times a week and he watched TV with her family. However, he started complaining that he could not hear his television programme while the family were talking, which ended up with Patricia mildly rebuking him. But it was the way in which her father reacted to her challenge that made Patricia more aware of how he had changed from his younger days.

> 'I said, "Why do you come round here because you come round here for conversation. You have been on your own all day and watching the telly. You can't expect to come round," I said, "and people not to talk. You can't tell people to be quiet". And he said [in a quiet, meek voice] "I couldn't hear my telly shows". And I [high guilty-sounding laugh] felt really horrible. [In an even quieter, meeker voice] "But I couldn't hear my programmes" and I said, "Well you can see your programmes any time", and if that had been ten years ago, [strong voice] "Here I can tell you what you can do, you can fuck off". That way he's changed. He's got old is what I mean really.'

This interaction was poignant and there was a real sense of guilt from Patricia, which was reflected in her uncertain laugh. She was no longer able to interact with her father on the same level as they once did. The dynamics of the relationship had shifted from him being a dominant, forthright, and strong father figure, to being a meek and weak character. This was something which Patricia now has to come to terms with.

Role confusion also occurred for adult child caregivers particularly when there was an increase in the parent's levels of dependency and a shift in the reciprocal relationship that once existed. Coleen's (aged 45) story is an example of this. She was unmarried, child-free, and living alone in London with a career as a legal secretary and a mortgaged property of her own.

When her father first started to require care at home, he lived alone 200 miles away, with failing health and onset dementia. As an only child her extended family expected her (and told her) to sell her home, give up her career, and move back into the family home to care for her dad. The burden of expectation upon her was causing enormous distress and overwhelming anxiety. Her dad's level of care then intensified following a fall at home and he was admitted to hospital. Coleen recalls how a social worker put an end to those caregiving pressures by suggesting that her dad should go into a care home when he left hospital. She remembers that the social worker told her "You still have to have your life." Coleen recalls:

> 'I was really grateful to that the social worker. They have such a bad press, and yet here he was putting my needs first, and I actually burst into tears. It was a relief, and I am ashamed to say this, and I will say this, but it almost felt like a get out of jail free card because I was about to become imprisoned as a carer. That's how I felt.'

Coleen lacked an adequate support system to help her transition into a caregiving role for her father. She was geographically distant from her dad and although she did travel to see him every week, she could not be with him every day to attend to his intensifying care needs. The extended family was unwilling and unable to help, and there was mounting pressure on her to relinquish her life and everything that was important to her in order to provide care. These familial expectations and her reluctance to give up everything to care for her dad only reinforced her sense of shame and guilt.

Caregiving role and physical health

Providing care which enables a parent to continue living independently in their own home can be a monumental task. Family members who provide care to older parents are at a greater risk of experiencing health problems themselves, including exhaustion, weakened immunity, anxiety, and depression (Gonyea et al, 2008, p 559). In Gonyea et al's (2008) study into 'Adult Daughters and Their Ageing Mothers' they found that three-quarters (74 per cent) of the daughters identified some level of burden as a result of becoming a carer for their mothers. For approximately 40 per cent the burden was either minimal (20 per cent) or moderate (20 per cent) while for 34 per cent the burden was either high (23 per cent) or very high (11 per cent) (Gonyea et al, 2008, p 563). The negative effects of caregiving can also result in higher levels of social isolation, physical and mental ill-health, and financial hardship (Brodaty and Donkin, 2009, p 217).

Unpaid care has been associated with lower levels of reported well-being including psychological distress, poorer physical health, strain on personal finances, difficulties in maintaining social relationships, stress on work life and educational opportunities, and an impact on the everyday activities of the carer. With intensive caring duties there is little time for socialising or even continuing life as normal. Furthermore, many of those caring for older parents have health conditions or disabilities themselves. Paoletti (2002, p 814) writes that 'Female caregivers often endanger their health carrying out caregiving tasks, mainly because they identify with their caring duties and see their social and moral meaning threatened by doing less'. Carers UK (2015) report that one in five people aged 50–64 are carers in the UK, but Age UK (2019) report that there are over 2 million carers aged over 65 and 417,000 of these are aged over 80. Older carers are also amongst those most likely to care at higher levels of intensity too (Age UK, 2019). When researching in care homes, I met relatives who were in their 80s with parents who were over 100 years old. In this case the adult child was older than some of the other residents in the care home. Adult children are themselves sometimes in poor health and struggle to visit.

Hazel (aged 68) remembers the exhaustion she felt following her caregiving experience for her mum. She told me wearily, "I feel structurally tired if you know what I mean?" When describing her experience, she said, "I started to feel desperate. I started to, I heard myself saying, in my head, 'How long can this go on for? Because I can't keep going on like this'." Hazel spoke about how she was unable to get close to her ageing aunt in her later years because she was still overwhelmed from caring for her mum. Alison (aged 63) also said, "Caring for mum was so tiring. You don't sleep well and that makes you even more tired. We never resented it, but I found it hard. Looking back, you wouldn't have wanted it any other way, but at the time it was so tiring."

Some tasks, such as attempting to lift a parent to assist in their mobility, can lead to physical strain and injury amongst untrained informal caregivers. Some adult child carers reported adverse physical issues as a result of their caring role, including changes to sleep patterns, inability to concentrate, of having a feeling that their head was too full, forgetting words, anxiety, and things feeling like more of an effort. Anxiety was a prevalent emotion amongst adult child participants in the research.

Trina (aged 70) was interviewed with her mother in a care home. Trina candidly said that before her mum moved into care, "I was going downhill rapidly. I did my back in humping a wheelchair around, you know it was hard." Coleen (aged 45) developed urge incontinence as a result of the stress of caring for her father. Some participants also began to catastrophise their own health, with stress symptoms being potentially indicative of something more ominous. Lily (aged 57) said that as a result of looking after her mum she was getting headaches and frightened about what these might mean. She said, "My head was sort of buzzing and aching. Then I got these sort of flashing things around my eyes, so I decided I was going blind." Sharon (aged 54) also recalled how physically and mentally stressful the situation was leading up to her mother's move into care. She remembered:

> 'I suppose a couple of years, year and a half, up to her going in the home, I was just stressed all the time. Really bad tempered. It was very, very stressful. So, at the point she went in, I just thought, you know, "I'm just going to have a heart attack or have a stroke or something. I'm just not going to be able to survive this."'

She went on to say:

> 'I feel like, for the last couple of years I've had no time for myself, so in ways of not eating properly, which is obviously affecting my health, and the stress levels and things, so I feel my health has deteriorated. I've noticed that my own health and my just general fitness has declined. I'm very aware of it, but I can't seem to do anything about it.'

At the time of interview, Sharon had just taken a sabbatical from work, so she could return to the gym and focus on regaining some level of fitness, as well as do some volunteering to recover her mental focus.

The pressures upon adult children can be overwhelming and can have adverse consequences. There are competing demands from multiple directions – children, career, own psychical and mental health, marriage, managing a home and the affairs of a parent's home, as well as loss, grief, and anxiety about a parent's ageing, choosing a care home, coping with guilt, as well as arbitrating other family and sibling relationships. It is perhaps not a surprise that some of the care home residents I spoke to said that their middle-aged children had recently died. This is discussed in more depth in Chapter 5, 'Social connections and relationship building in residential care'.

Intimate bonds

As a parent's assistance needs increase in old age, the caregiving process becomes more intense. And whereas some more informative or instrumental care tasks, like speaking to a GP, cleaning, or making a hot meal may have been anticipated care tasks, there is sometimes a shift to more unanticipated care duties. One of the most challenging and often unanticipated aspects of providing care for an older parent concerns attending to a parent's intimate, personal care needs. Lily (aged 57) tells her story of how her anticipated care duties became an experience of unanticipated intimate care:

> 'I used to go around at least once a week. I used to go in every Saturday morning, and do things like checking the fridge, and making her some

lunch, and sometimes I'd take her out. Then there was one time when I just realised that she'd stopped having showers, and it was either because she'd forgotten, or she didn't want to get cold, or she was scared of slipping, or I don't know exactly what, but I thought, "She's going to have to have a shower," you know, "She just can't not shower!" I went in with her. I tried to help her, and it was just appalling. It was appalling on so many fronts, and I was so scared that I was going to burn her, but I didn't. It was the proximity, you know, everything was just … I mean, maybe some people could do that and would be fine with it, but I just couldn't. So, then we started getting carers coming in, and that was such a battle. She used to phone and cancel them, and say "I don't need them", and "It's a waste of money", and "I don't want them in my house", but we just kind of made it work eventually.'

Lily also had to have a difficult conversation about incontinence with her mum. She said:

'My younger sister was the one that said, "Oh well, we'll just have to talk to her about incontinence pads", but at the time I was like, "You can't say that!". And I think that's a real hotspot for people because I know I've heard people saying, "Oh, I can't put him in nappies", and that's the real role reversal thing, isn't it? It's really, really, really difficult. But my mother was so relieved that somebody had said something.'

Other participants described providing physical, intimate care for a parent and described it as like looking after a child. Hazel (aged 68) said, "When somebody is dependent on you, the relationship changes. You know, it felt like having a child, wiping her bottom."

Although much of the existing literature has focused upon caregiver burden, there is also evidence of some positive dimensions to caregiving and evidence of caregiver growth (Roberto and Jarrott, 2008). Despite the challenges of caring for a parent, it can also be incredibly rewarding and a special period of bonding. It can also be associated with personal fulfilment and satisfaction. Roberto and Jarrott (2008, p 103) recognised positive dimensions of the caregiving experience, such as the 'development of competence, or an individual's sense of ability in the role (Pearlin et al, 1990), coping skills that enhance caregiver ability, and fulfilment in the caregiving role'. Miller et al (2008, p 22) recognised rewards in the caregiving experience, such as personal satisfaction, increased sense of purpose in life, companionship, and overall well-being. And Brodaty and Donkin (2009, p 218) reported that the majority of caregivers experienced 'positive experiences such as enjoying togetherness, sharing activities, feeling a reciprocal bond, spiritual and personal growth, increased faith, and feelings of accomplishments and mastery'.

Providing intimate, personal care can be a bonding experience as it requires new levels of trust, touch, and connection. Sharon (aged 54) recalled how the experience had transformed a previously strained relationship with her mother to one of love and connection which they were unable to find through other means. Sharon had described their relationship prior to her mum's dementia, saying "We didn't have a great relationship. She wasn't much of a 'mumsy' kind of mum, do you know what I mean? She was quite selfish as a person really." She continued, "She had a bit of a nasty streak in her which seems to have gone, which is so weird!" Sharon had initially struggled with what to do on visits to the care home to see her mum but found that playing an active role in her personal care was one way of them reconnecting.

> '[Mum] said "Oh, I wouldn't do this in front of anyone else" and "It's fantastic of you". "It's really good of you to do it, I'll give you 2/6d!", like she always makes a joke of it! She's able to wash herself, but she doesn't like a shower, and she can't get in the bath – physically, she can't get in the bath. So, they have their little shower room in their en-suite. And there's an assisted bath with a hydraulic chair, so after a while I persuaded her to do it with me. She still doesn't let the carers do it, but she'll let me help her have a bath. I do that once a week and make sure she's cleaned her teeth, because she hides her toothbrush. I can't ask them to make sure she cleans her teeth, they've got enough to do, so at least I know she's done it once a week! [Laughs]. She doesn't look like she's not well-kept or well looked after. That might take two hours to have a bath because she messes around – she won't be in the bath for two hours, but she messes around, and the getting there, and getting out. But I quite like that because it's something to do. And she talks to me when she's in the bath, and she's generally very light-hearted and jokes a lot and stuff. I mean, I find it quite depressing just sitting in the lounge with her.'

She now cherishes the time she shares with her mum in the care home now and finds that they have developed a more intimate bond. Being able to reciprocate care to a parent, who spent time caring for them as a child, was an important experience of affection for many of the participants.

Chapter summary

Informal caregivers play a critical role in the social care system, but the impact upon them is often underestimated, undervalued, and goes unrecognised, not only within family systems, but also by wider policy makers. Coming to recognise that a parent requires increasing care can be frightening, overwhelming, and disorientating, and adult children experience changes in the relationship with their parents, shifts in their own role identity, and reawakened sibling dynamics as they negotiate their emerging caregiving role.

This chapter has shown how a shift in role identity from son or daughter to 'carer' can be difficult to come to terms with and can challenge the adult child's self-perception, and their relationships with their parents. Equally, once that label of 'carer' has been adopted, there may well be a shift back to being a 'son' or 'daughter' again once the older parent has transitioned into care, which can be equally hard to come to terms with. It is important here for adult children to recognise that their caring role can continue once their parent is in a care home, and for care staff to enable adult children to continue care giving roles should they be desired.

We have seen how caring for a parent is something that often emerges over a period of time, unless there is a catastrophic health event. And the experience of caring is a relational and ongoing construction, which is fluid and dynamic dependent upon the care receiver's needs and the caregiver's ability to attend to those needs. In the context of cognitive impairment through dementia, there may be drastic changes in the older person's personality which changes the relationship they have with their adult children. As we have seen in this chapter, this can be for the worse or for the better.

The change in family dynamics was another important part of caring for a parent and this was most evident in sibling groups. Siblings often negotiate among themselves as to who will provide what form of care, with sisters often taking on more of the emotional caregiving tasks, and brothers managing instrumental tasks; historic dynamics emerging as brothers and sisters try to coordinate and distribute caregiving roles.

Finally, this chapter considered the definition of care as multi-dimensional, involving a range of task-based activities which are often over-laid with an emotional charge. There were complex motives for why children take on care roles for their ageing parents. Some adult children felt a sense of obligation, originating from their own moral judgement, from the expectations put upon them by family members or from (particularly gendered) societal expectations. Some cared for their older parents out of love, respect, and wanting to reciprocate the early experiences of care that they received. And some care for parents at home for as long as possible due to fears about what a move into the care system might mean. In the next chapter we will explore further the care trajectories that older adults follow leading up to admission into a care facility, the complexity of care options, and how the whole process is emotionally navigated by adult children and their older parents as they face one of the most significant events in their lives.

3

The transition to care

Making the decision – for and with older parents – to transition into residential care is fraught with challenges. The move to long-term care is often preceded by a sudden health crisis, a deterioration of an existing condition, and the inability for care to be provided at home any longer. Choosing which home is right for the older person is a complicated process with multiple factors to consider: What type of care is right for my older parent and how might their care requirements change over time? What is the cost and how will we finance it? How will the home cater to my parent's individual interests and needs? Will the staff love and care for my parent? And after all that consideration, do they even have a vacancy? Adult children and their older parents are challenged by all these questions and many more, and all within the context of pervasive negative stereotypes about what care will actually be like.

The focus of this chapter is on older parents who have lived in their own homes and who are now transitioning into long-term residential care. It considers a range of trajectories into care that older people might take, including falls or sudden health crises, more gradual declines in cognition, and loneliness and bereavement. Participants for my studies were sampled based on them having a parent move into a residential care home, so although alternative arrangements for care such as moving in with children or moving to sheltered housing were discussed in family conversations, they were decided against amongst this research population. We will hear the voices of adult children and their decision-making processes, as well as the voices of older adults whose voices have typically not been heard or are often not taken into account when planning transitions to care.

Care options

In the UK there are a wide variety of long-term care (LTC) options for older people. The most common include the following: *Retirement communities*, which tend to accommodate retirees who all live in the same area. These communities of older residents often have a sense of collectivity and mutual interests, and the housing arrangement provides them with a sense of autonomy and at the same time a sense of mutual support, safety, and security. *Domiciliary care* is a type of care which provides support to someone in their own home, enabling them to remain independent in their own environment for as long as possible. *Sheltered housing* is accommodation where older adults can live in a specific complex of separate houses, which are all centrally maintained and often have a warden on call in case of emergencies. *Assisted living housing* is similar but has the addition of a central dining space and sometimes housekeeping services too. *Extra care housing* is an extension of these forms of shelter but includes adaptations for major disabilities and provides nursing care on site. *Residential care homes* provide housing with full board, all maintenance and housekeeping, and 24-hour care for those with significant physical and/or cognitive disabilities. Around 70 per cent of care homes are residential and around 29 per cent are *nursing homes* (carehome. co.uk, 2022). These two types of residential care share similarities, but nursing homes provide additional complex medical care for more advanced physical and mental disabilities (Westwood and Daly, 2016, p 12). All the adult child relatives interviewed for these studies were sampled on the basis that they made decisions to move their parent into a *residential care home*.

Older people may follow a 'housing trajectory' which follows their changing care needs and financial resources, and these factors can lead to 'voluntary or involuntary moves to different housing in later life' (Westwood and Daly, 2016, p 15). For example, an older person may begin with domiciliary care providing support in their own home, but when this no longer provides enough support, they may move to a residential home, and finally onto a different nursing home if specialist medical treatment is required and cannot be provided at the residential home. The average life expectancy in UK care homes is 24 months for care homes without nursing care, and 12 months for care homes with nursing support (British Geriatrics Society, 2020).

In addition to the different types of care support, care facilities and providers can be variable in scale, provision, and in the way they are funded. The majority of care homes are run by private organisations. These can range in size from small properties with one or two residents to national organisations with thousands of residents across multiple homes. There are also care homes run by charities and voluntary organisations, and only a relatively small proportion of care homes are provided by local authorities. Instead, local authorities generally tend to commission care services from private care providers. The 'Adult Social Care Market in England' report by the Department for Health and Social Care (2021) states that '76% of care homes for older adults and adults with dementia are for-profit. Of the remaining 24%, 14% are not-for-profit and 10% are run by a local authority or the NHS'. The care homes sector is said to have an estimated worth of £15.9 billion per year, across 11,300 care homes for older people in the UK (CMA, 2017). There are some residents who self-fund their care, and others who are state funded, both often living within one care facility.

With such complexities in the care market, it is not surprising that there is competition and debate over which provision is best for older people. There are stereotypes which characterise these discussions: 'the public sector seen as bureaucratic and wasteful, or reliable and dependable; whilst the private sector is seen as lean, innovative and customer-centric or as self-serving and profit-driven (Powell and Miller, 2013)' (Hall et al, 2016, p 540). Hall et al also report differences between these various forms of provision, including 'staff job satisfaction, motivation and commitment; clientele characteristics; organizational goals and performance; and levels of organizational red tape (Anderson, 2013; Bozeman and Moulton, 2011; Walker and Bozeman, 2011; Rainey and Bozeman, 2000)' (2016, p 542). Regardless of the provider, all care homes are regularly inspected for quality by the Care Quality Commission (CQC) which independently regulates health and social care across England. The CQC inspects, regulates, and takes action where it is needed. Comprehensive inspections are conducted to ensure that 'services are providing care that's safe, caring, effective, responsive to people's needs and well-led' (Care Quality Commission, 2022). The CQC also publish reports and ratings to help those looking for care make informed choices about their care.

The perception of care homes

Concerns about moving into a care home often stem from unhelpful and undermining stereotypes that care homes are places of loneliness, isolation, and inadequate care, representative of suffering, dying and loss.

One of the primary indicators of perceived poor care amongst the adult children that I interviewed was the smell of the home, with one of the key deciding factors on choosing a care facility being that the home 'didn't smell of urine'. A care home manager even encouraged relatives to use a sense of smell to help make a decision. She said:

> 'You can go into the most fantastic buildings with everything, you know, high quality furniture and chandeliers and everything else, but it, it's not that, I mean, it's nice, but it's not that that you should be looking at. And use your nose! Because if a home doesn't smell nice, there's a problem.'

Jilly (aged 68) outlined the factors she was considering when looking at care home options for her mum. I asked, "was there anything in particular you were looking for when you were going round the different homes? What were you looking out for?" She replied:

> 'Oh well, the atmosphere. Straight away, I think it sort of hits you what a place is like. This has a really good atmosphere, and it doesn't smell of anything bad. No, I mean, it doesn't necessarily in many homes, but in one I went to, that one had a terrible smell of urine in it. Somebody

had obviously made a mistake and peed, which can happen to anybody, but it just put me off! And there was also some screaming going on. Again, it was probably an off day, but screaming, I mean, I've never ever heard anything like that here. I mean, it's probably occurred, and I haven't been here, of course, because everyone's human. Something might have happened to someone here that I'm just not aware of. But, but the, but the atmosphere of that place wasn't good, and here, I knew the atmosphere is very good. And so, I think you look for the light of the atmosphere, and people, and lightness, do you know what I mean?'

Jilly's experience of visiting a home was quite confronting. For those who have never visited a care home setting before, the sight of advanced agedness, bodily decline, and extreme frailty can really bring to the fore their own parent's ageing and may also serve as a reminder about their own mortality. Whitaker (2009, p 160) writes about family involvement in choosing nursing care, that 'seeing all the frailty clearly tended to arouse anxiety among the relatives about their own prospective ageing and dying'. She continues, 'residents, staff and visiting relatives all had different names for it, but the meaning was the same; this is a place where old people come to die' (Whitaker, 2009, p 160). Workers in nursing and the care sector may become accustomed to bodily functions and secretions, deteriorating and dying bodies, but relatives and visitors to care homes may never have encountered such sights and smells, and this can have a profound impact upon them. One of the unfortunate consequences is that this can result in inexperienced staff and unsupported volunteers leaving abruptly. One care home volunteer, who I was observing, left her role after just three visits saying:

'To be honest I was very surprised at how poorly some of the residents were when I was given a tour of the home. I suppose I was expecting elderly people who were just in need of some company. I spent some time there for a couple of weeks but to be honest I was just left to "get on with it" and went to a couple of rooms to talk to people but found it quite upsetting that unfortunately most of them had dementia. Again, I was very naive I think. I am sure that my dad passing away had something to do with this decision. He was very healthy and aware of everything, and I found it terribly upsetting that these people were in such a sad way.'

Care homes are sites of ambiguity: death and dying contradicted by life and care. Staff are required in their everyday work roles to manage complex needs, frailty, and death. On a wider societal level, anxiety about how dying and older bodies are managed is often translated to a policy level of 'we need to sort these homes out', which can lead to an attack or bombardment of measures on the home. The homes then do not always feel they have the backing of policy makers and unfortunately a consequence of this is that abuse in care homes occurs when homes feel under attack and secret themselves away. My Home Life England, however, has been working really hard to change this negative stereotype of care homes. Founded in 2006, My Home Life England is a UK-wide initiative that seeks to promote quality of life and deliver positive change in care homes for older people by identifying and sharing best practice, focusing on the positive relationships involved in care, and promoting an appreciative approach to understanding care provision (My Home Life England, 2022). They state that 'My Home Life wanted to focus more positively on care homes, sharing best practice and inspirational stories of success' (My Home Life England, 2022). It advocates for appreciative enquiry, which is a process of noticing and asking 'What is working now and what more do we need to do to make it even better?' (My Home Life England, 2022). The My Home Life England movement challenges the current regulatory and persecutory practices of uncovering the negative side of care by working with the principle of 'appreciative enquiry', focusing on the good work that care homes do so that it might set a standard and a model for others to follow.

Care trajectories

In my research, there were powerful narratives from older people and adult children about the journey into residential care. Some were stories of dramatic and traumatic moves, and others were stories of resistance and relationship breakdowns. Others were stories of loss, and some were stories of relief and finally feeling safe. Each older person follows their own unique trajectory into care.

Glaser and Strauss (1968), in their classic treatise on death, write about dying trajectories. Dying trajectories include the duration (the length of the dying course) and shape (the slope of individuals' decline as they approach death). These dying trajectories can be sudden or span days, months, or years (Ball et al, 2014). There are similar trajectories which lead into long-term care. The transition to care can include a gradual decline associated with advancing age and chronic conditions, or a steep decline relating to terminal diagnoses, and a rapid trajectory resulting from a sudden crisis such as a fall or accident. The three most common pathways into care identified across my research related to falls and sudden health crises, cognitive decline, and loneliness, which will be the focus here.

Falls

For many older parents in this study, having a fall began their trajectory into care. Even if the fall did not result in serious injury, the concerns about their safety were heightened. Falls can have a significant impact upon the older person's confidence, independence, and overall well-being. When the older person's confidence is affected in such a way following a fall, this may be the moment they ask for further help or ask to move into care even after a period of resistance. For example, Diana (aged 99) recalled "I was in my own home. I did live alone. My daughter, she found me on the floor twice 'that's it!' and I said, 'oh put me in somewhere'."

Rapid trajectories into care often followed a fall, particularly when they resulted in broken bones – typically broken hips – and falls were sometimes the result of a stroke. Having a fall in later life that results in a prolonged hospital stay increases the time spent sedentary which in turn increases the risk of muscle weakness and consequent falls (Arora, 2017). Falls and hospital stays can also accelerate cognitive decline, meaning that, in combination with limited mobility, independent living is no longer possible. This move from hospital direct to care was usually decided by health and social care professionals who took over the difficult decision-making process, releasing the adult child from that responsibility.

Cognitive decline

Gradual, but more common, trajectories into care were the result of cognitive decline. The Alzheimer's Society UK report that 70 per cent of people in care homes have dementia or severe memory problems. Dementia is an umbrella term for a range of progressive, terminal conditions that affect the brain (Dementia UK, 2019). Alzheimer's disease is the most common type of dementia and affects between 60-80% of those diagnosed (World Health Organisation, 2023).

A route to care as a result of dementia is often preceded by fluctuating and contested meanings attributed by adult children to new behaviours displayed by their older parent. The symptoms of dementia are primarily emotional and behavioural rather than physical, and thus can cause contention in identifying and defining what is actually happening. Dementia can cause impairment in emotional regulation and cognition. Symptoms can include memory loss and misidentification; depression and changes in mood or personality, with behavioural problems such as agitation, disorientation, inhibition, and aggression; impaired judgement, which can lead to difficulties in making complex decisions; difficulty in communicating or expressing themselves; and sleep disturbance. With the progression of the condition the person will require help with the activities of daily living. It should be noted, however, that not all these symptoms are present in all cases. Adult children spoke about how they found themselves confused by early displays of out-of-character behaviour. Over time, they learned to recognise the early signs of dementia and the associated behaviours. It was when they were unable to justify or normalise these behaviours that they were able to recognise that they needed external support and sought diagnosis. Lily (aged 57) recalled that the alarming early signs of her mother's dementia:

> 'We were all at hers for some reason and she said something and then she said exactly the same thing a minute later, and that was just weird, because, you know, people repeat themselves and they tell stories, but they just, it was like, "But you just said that", and she didn't say, "Oh, did I just say that?" No, she just said it again. And there was just a moment of "That's weird. That's weird".'

Over time, Lily's mother would call to ask how to switch the iron on, the house became unkempt, and Lily would find things around her mum's house which were out of place. Then her mum started to forget things, leaving her purse in a shop, or forgetting her keys. Noticing the signs of decline in her mum's cognitive health resulted in a formal diagnosis.

> 'She slowly, slowly, slowly, just sort of, you know, we just noticed things weren't right. We'd talk about it, and "What can we do?" and, "What's going on?" And then eventually we got her to the doctor and then to the Memory Clinic and when she was diagnosed and they used "dementia" and "Alzheimer's" fairly interchangeably, and it was like a brick had landed on my head. The only thing I knew about Alzheimer's then was that film with Iris Murdoch, which I saw, ironically, with my mother, and she always used to say, "If I get like that, put a pillow over my head", so it was a real, real shock. As it turns out she's still not that bad today, but at the time it was such a shock.'

With Lily's mum previously telling her to put a 'pillow over my head' if she was to develop dementia, Lily found herself in a challenging position. Obviously, this was not an option Lily would ever even consider for her mum, but she was left in a quandary about how to care for a parent with dementia who has previously held such pessimistic views about her potential for quality of life. How could she positively support her mum when she knew her mum would not want to live with this condition? Lily noticed that her mother's condition would worsen in the evenings, and she would receive worrying phone calls from her mum.

> 'I think, generally, with Alzheimer's, quite often they get this "Sundowners" thing. By the end of the day, they get more tired, and more confused, and they have hallucinations. When she was at home, I mean, that, that, was also very scary, you know, she'd phone up and say, "Oh, there's somebody in the flat", and I'd think, "Oh, my God!

Who's in the flat?" And then sometimes she'd say, "Oh I've been playing cards with my dad", or something, and that's sort of quite spooky. But she has stopped doing that (since moving into care) because I think she's just more secure, stable, and she's eating properly, and she's got somebody keeping an eye on her.'

These experiences left Lily on edge all the time, wondering what the next phone call would be and whether her mum was safe or not. Lily and her siblings started to plan their mother's care and considered whether their mum could move in with any of them, or if any of them could move in with her. But then their mum went missing on a 'boiling hot day' whilst wearing a winter coat and when discovered was found to be overheated. Lily recalled that that was the moment when they thought "That's it! We'll have to do something" and they decided that she would be safer in a care home.

Sharon (aged 54) had had a really difficult and fractious relationship with her mum for a long period of time leading up to her diagnosis and move into care. Like Lily, Sharon first noticed a change in her mum's behaviour when she was repeating herself and not fully understanding what was being said: "She would say 'what are you doing tonight?', and I'd tell her, and she'd ask me 20 times." She would get off the tube and go in the wrong direction when meeting her daughter at a regular stop. And she would frequently be late, but then blame her daughter for her tardiness. At home, Sharon noticed that things were becoming untidy, and washing loads had increased. She remembered:

'It kind of went, because you don't really know what's wrong with a person, then you suddenly, things, – especially if you're not living there – suddenly things make sense. Like there was always so much washing, and, and I realised it was because she was soiling all her clothes, and, you know, she was still able to put them in the washing machine and put the washing on, but she said, "There's always so much washing everywhere.'

When Sharon was clearing her mum's house, following her move into care, she found notes which her mum had written to herself which said, "heart-breaking stuff, things that were saying 'I think I'm losing my mind'". Like Lily's mum, Sharon's mum also started suffering from hallucinations. "She had a dream that my dad was in the house, and I realise, now, that that must have been a hallucination, because she was really disturbed by him. She used to think I was still there when I wasn't there, and that kind of stuff." Seeing figures in her house was really disturbing for Sharon and she didn't know how to support her through these experiences.

Hazel spoke about how, when her mum was 96, she began to forget things and was eventually diagnosed with Alzheimer's. The medication she was initially given had such negative side-effects – including sweating, shaking, nightmares, and insomnia – that Hazel and her mother jointly agreed that she should stop taking the medication. Hazel recalled that "She didn't recognise that she needed to put knickers on, or she'd get up at three o'clock in the morning and get dressed, put things over her nightie. I couldn't move in there. I could have, but I didn't want to." Hazel's house was open plan, and it felt unsafe for her mum to move in with her, both physically and emotionally for the both of them. She said:

> 'Well, even if I'd put a bed here, she'd have to go up to the loo. She could do that in her own home – have banisters both sides – and she was used to it. Right? I didn't really want to. I did think about it, and I dismissed it immediately. I could not see myself as a 24-hour carer. I thought she'd be safer, actually, in all sorts of ways, physically safer, and I didn't want to get to a stage where I was getting miserable, she'd be safer that way too, you know.'

Hazel visited her mum up to three times a day before she moved into the care home, helping with mealtimes, or just simply sitting and holding her hand. Her mum began attending a day centre, and participated in singing, painting, and reading activities there, but as her Alzheimer's progressed she was no longer able to take part. Hazel remembers that the day centre said to her, "There's not much point in her coming, she might as well sit at home", and she replied "No, because she's with people". Hazel eventually called a local care home, and a social worker came round and told them that it was perhaps time to move.

Loneliness

Loneliness is another important factor in the trajectory into care. Older people are more at risk of loneliness and a reduction in meaningful interactions and conversations. Age UK (2021) note that 'loneliness can have a significant impact on older people's health and well-being and is associated with worse physical and mental health in older people'. This became an increasing problem during the COVID-19 pandemic due to shielding and the inability to interact with friends and family during this period.

When I interviewed Trina (aged 70) with her mother Diana, Trina was visibly upset by the trauma and the deep feelings of guilt for moving her mother into a care home. Diana was almost 100 years old and had had two falls. Trina said her mum had been "staring at four walls with only the TV for company". Diana said, "I lived alone. I used to talk to the wall, talk to anything." Trina suggested her mum went into respite in the home for two weeks and at that visit her mum had decided she really wanted to stay there because she had had such a good time. Trina recalls, "That was all she had, four walls and a television … she was just not mixing with people and went very into herself, very, very into herself." She continued, "The telly was her life, there was nothing else but the television, but here she doesn't even bother to watch it!"

The television is a lifeline for many older people. It provides older people with company, entertainment, a source of comfort, and information about the wider world. During the pandemic it became even more important. Caroline Abrahams, Charity Director at Age UK (2020), stated that 'TV is extremely important to many older people at the happiest of times, but it has taken on a whole new meaning at this time of danger and crisis, when access to authoritative information matters so much'. However, because the television is so important in the lives of older people, when technology changes or the television doesn't work, this can be a source of great distress. For example, when I interviewed Rob (aged 50) we were interrupted by a phone call from his 79-year-old mother who has dementia. It was evident from the call that his mother was in great distress and urgently wanted him to go to her, but despite this he waved off the urgency and insisted we continued with the interview. When we had finished, he said, "Yeah, I better had go see my mum." He said about the call, "There is that transition now, we had a phone call just a few minutes ago, she can't put the TV on so whose responsibility is it to sort it out? It's mine." Rob would then need to travel about an hour to his mum's house to turn her television on before returning home again late in the evening. I wondered whether his mother had called him in part about the television, but also due to her increasing loneliness which she had been struggling with since the death of her husband (Rob's father). Rob described her as "a very lonely lady" and he had been looking into care options for her as a result of her decreasing mental health, exacerbated by her situation of isolated living.

Loneliness usually follows the death of a spouse in later life. Age UK report that 'The average age of being widowed is around 73 for women and 77 for men' (2019, p 2) and that 'bereavement is a major cause of loneliness and isolation' (2019, p 3). Many of the older people whom I interviewed in the care homes had suffered the death of their spouse, and even if they had – up until that point – been coping at home with a physical health condition, this was the event that expedited their transition to care.

Moving in with family

Despite issues of loneliness and bereavement, older parents were often reluctant to move in with family members and these arrangements do not always work out if they do go ahead. 'An older adult may enjoy ongoing, regular contact with their adult children, yet living with them is not usually desired and does not usually alleviate loneliness' (Hagan et al, 2020, p 277). Shanas (1979, p 170, in Hagan et al, 2020, p 277) wrote that the favoured position of older people was for 'intimacy at a distance'. Moving in with an adult child can help provide practical support, social contact, and address some health-care needs. However, these factors can be negated by reduced privacy, dependency, lack of autonomy, fears of becoming a burden, and sometimes family conflict. Hagan et al (2020, p 284) write:

> Living with adult children may help address certain social needs and practical forms of support but cannot salve the yearnings of emotional loneliness. It may be that a crisis, which may be a painful transition such as a bereavement, or sudden health decline, leads to a living arrangement, which is simultaneously helpful and protective, while also imbued with loss, a sense of helplessness and other negative emotions. (Robinson and Stell, 2015)

Many of the adult children I interviewed had given serious thought to the more intense personal care that their parents might require in the future. Most were not keen to take on the caring role and were even less enthusiastic about inviting older parents to live with them at home. Joe (aged 49), for instance, said, "Oh I could never have had mum in the house. No way." Thirty-nine-year-old Sarah said, "I couldn't give up my life to look after parents." When I asked Fred (aged 56) whether he had considered his parents coming to live with him, he replied, "I think we've probably talked about it and dismissed it probably within about five minutes. Literally! Even if you love them, and they were your mum and dad, and they looked after you when you were small, you can buy yourself out of that." It was also difficult or awkward for children to turn away parents who asked to live with them. Kathleen (aged 46), for example, said, "My dad's made a few, couple of flippant comments before now like 'Oh, when we sell our house, we'll move in with you' and I think 'No, no don't go there!'"

Older parents, too, worried about the impact on their families if they were to move in and they did not want to become a burden to them. Some of the older people I interviewed recognised that there might be tensions and conflict at home, should they move in with their children. Care home resident Jessie (aged in her 80s) said "That's when trouble starts when you move in with family. However much they love you, you're under their feet."

Discussing a move into care

Talking to parents about the move into care can be fraught with difficulties and tensions, and, depending on the circumstances, older parents may or may not be included in the decision-making processes about where they might move to.

Some adult children found it impossible to involve their parents in the decision-making process due to their cognitive decline. Alison (aged 63) recalled "We'd been trying, trying, and trying and trying to persuade her she needed more help in that sort of way in that last year. But she was a very stubborn lady!" Her mum would say, " 'Oh no, dear. I'm all right, dear' ", Alison said, "She was quite convinced she was going to get better." Lily (aged 57) described how her mum "Just didn't want to talk about it" or plan anything. Lord et al (2016, p 2) found in a recent systematic literature review that 'family carers find proxy decision-making, especially around place of care, challenging and distressing, especially when decisions are made against the wishes of the care recipient and support from health-care professionals is lacking'. I found that some adult child relatives resorted to telling 'little white lies' in order to transition their parent into care. Sharon (aged 54), for example, told how she persuaded her mum to move from hospital into a care home just for 'convalescence'. She said her mum was "very aggressive, and very against it" but she would constantly have to reassure her mum that it was 'only temporary' when in reality her mum's house had to be sold without her knowledge to pay for the care. One care home manager remembered a similar case, where the resident "had to be told a version of the story that isn't totally the truth, and – to make it better for her".

Some of the older people I interviewed did not feel like they were part of the decision-making process but were happy for their family to take charge. Joy (aged in her 80s) remembered, "The family got together and got me here. And it's the best thing that's ever happened to me." Betty (aged 86) felt she had a small part to play in the decision about where she moved to: "I got a list, and I was told I couldn't go home. I got a list of houses or places that I could go and see and pick the one I wanted."

Coleen's story

Coleen (aged 45) was a single, child-free woman, who lived alone in London in her own home and had a thriving career as a legal secretary. She was an only child, her mother died aged 62 and her dad, aged 74, now had advanced dementia. Her dad's decline in health began with a "funny turn" on the way to church when he collapsed in the street as a result of a mini stroke. She describes this as "The beginning of the nightmare really because he never went home again." Initially her dad suffered physical injuries as a result of the fall, injuring his face and shoulder, but she said "It was as if the dementia was waiting in the background, thinking, 'Right! Here's my opportunity', and after only a couple of weeks, suddenly the deterioration kicked in so fast." She described his decline as "huge and dramatic". She began to notice a decline in his personal hygiene. He had stopped washing, his hair had become greasy, and he stopped cleaning his house. She describes these as seemingly all "very, very minor things" but they rapidly became really concerning. She remembered:

'It was the saddest thing. I came up on a Saturday to see my dad and I suddenly noticed he'd stopped preparing food, and he'd obviously gone down to the local supermarket, he'd bought all his vegetables as he always did, and just, overnight, stopped cooking, and they were all in the pantry, all going mouldy. There was indication that this was going to happen, it just happened. And my dad was starving. He wasn't really hungry. I said, "Dad, have you, you've not eaten?" And he was just like, "No", and he had all this food.'

She recalls finding out that social services were really keen on him staying at home with a package of care in place to support his needs.

Relatives on both sides of her family had had an expectation that she would care for her father in later life "Because I'm the daughter. I don't have children. I'm the perfect solution." The family network all expected her to give up life to look after him – "everyone expected me to do that". She remembers thinking:

'Yeah, that's the obvious solution. It's what I need to do. It's my duty, I have to do it. But I was terrified! I was physically sick at the thought of it. Not just, not so much looking after my dad, but more the case of, "Well, how long could this go on for?" because this could go on for eight to ten years, and I am now 45. I shall be 55. Who will look after me? Who cares for the carer? How am I going to financially support myself? How would I get a job at 55? And I know that sounds brutal to be considering that when it was my dad who needed consideration, and I felt guilty for even considering that.'

She continued:

'The guilt is horrendous. It just, it just eats you up, you know. You do feel there must be something wrong with you because you're sort of terrified of taking on that role, and you're being selfish because you're looking at yourself as well, and you're weighing it all up. It's the most horrendous situation to be in. You go around and around and around, trying to find the right solution. And you think, "Right. Okay. If I move back and convert the downstairs for my dad, and maybe I'd be upstairs", because all my life I've been on my own, but not lonely. I really like my own space, and I left home at 17 and to suddenly move back in again, and then I think, "Well, stop being selfish. This is about your dad now. He went and did his horrible job, so you had a roof over your house, it's your turn to give back".'

Coleen's account highlights the obligations and expectations expressed within women's accounts of caregiving practices. She also indicates a sense of duty and a reciprocal exchange of care. This is the idea that it is now her turn to 'give back' but that she feels that she is failing in her inability to fulfil that duty. She said:

'My worst nightmare was me sort of putting my life on hold – and this sounds so brutal saying that – but the next stage was, "Right. Need to find the very best place for him". I don't have a car, "How am I going to drive around?" "Right, do I move him down to London where I am?" Dad always hated London, absolutely hated London with a passion.'

Coleen started to look around different care facilities. "I thought they were all horrendous! I mean, they're not horrendous, but just because of what they are. I was struggling to accept the reality of the situation" and "[I had] another burst into tears moment, it all just got a bit too much because I had to now make that decision, and I hated every one of them."

For Coleen, talking to her dad about his advancing dementia had been a traumatic experience, which threatened their relationship. She explained:

'I saw those adverts and I thought "It's time to face up to this now. I am going to have to have that conversation with dad" and that was horrible actually … I did phone him and I did say "Have you seen those adverts on TV? I think we need to talk about this. I am really sorry to have to use the 'D word' but I do think you've got [whispered] dementia" and he got really angry, and my dad doesn't get angry. He is so placid. He is so very, very placid but he actually did get angry, and he said to me [shouting] "I am disappointed in you". The conversation didn't end well. He was distraught.'

She continued, "[I said to him] 'I'm really sorry. I'm sorry I have to be the one to say it to you. No one else is going say it to you. You have to, we have to face up to this'. And [he replied] 'I'm disappointed with you. I'm disappointed you saying that'."

Adult children often feel very guilty about moving their parents into formal care and see it as a sign of weakness and failure if they cannot or will not care for their parents at home. When the chosen care home is not to the expected standard this can exacerbate the guilt and anxiety surrounding the decision. When Coleen's dad first moved into a care home, they both found the care to be substandard. She found that the rooms in his care home were not being heated properly and her dad was not being washed regularly, "the typical nightmare that you hope won't happen in a care home". She remembered: "I would go up and he would absolutely stink." She went on:

> 'The worst part was when I came up and his room was freezing cold, and I just said, "Right. I'm not happy with this", and "You just sort this out, or I'll make a call to social workers", and at the same time I started, again, that process of looking for alternative homes.'

She remembers how she felt like she became the "the bitch daughter" because she was always complaining to the care staff. She recalls how this made her feel, and how it made her reconsider her decisions about her dad's care. She said:

> 'When you come in and your dad is in an unheated room, and then you feel horrendous about that because that's a failure on your part. "I should be coming up there every day?", "I should take a sabbatical from work?" "Coming up once a week is not going be good enough in this situation".'

Eventually the care home took notice of her complaints and the manager's employment was terminated. She describes this management shift as being pivotal, "The home went from being a shocker to one of nicest, kindest places."

Moving into a care home

Older people living in care often expressed a sense of resignation and an understanding that they were being cared for in a way which couldn't happen or continue as it was before. Yet, moving into care necessarily involved loss and grief for lives that had to be left behind. Betty saw her move to care as a start of a new life and expressed a resignation to the change. She said, "This is a new life. But it, it's a job to come to that conclusion. It's not easy by any means. And at 86, I don't really want to start a new life." Almost all of the residents expressed a reluctance and a dislike of the home when they first moved in but went on to describe how they quickly settled and found positives in their new living arrangements. Elisabeth (aged 84) recalled how when she first arrived in the home she said "Oh, I don't like this" but how she "got used to it". Mildred (aged 86) was quite sad about the move and found it hard to accept that this was where she lived. She said, "It's not the sort of thing that you think you're going to end up in in life" and whilst she recognised that she needed the additional care that the home could provide, and needed the company of others, she still experienced a terrible sense of loss for the life she used to have. However, like many of the older people I interviewed there was a stoicism in their narratives. Mr Randall (aged 98) demonstrated a 'war spirit' in his move, saying "It didn't worry me. No, that's because I'd had six years in the war. We used to make a home wherever the convoy stopped. You'd learnt to do it, and that stood me in very good stead." Other narratives described a desire to look for the positives and avoid retrospection. Mildred said, "It's no good looking back, it doesn't do. Not really. It is sense to go, even if that's only for a little while, to go forwards." Betty found that looking forward was the only way that she could psychologically negotiate this transition. She said resolutely, "The past has got to go back" and "It's got to be a backdrop, if you like, in a play – like a backdrop when you're doing a play. I thought, 'That's got to go behind, and you've got to live for the future' and that is what I have tried to do."

Sometimes the move and associated losses reignited the memories of a late spouse, which compounded their grief. Elisabeth (aged 84) was married for 56 years to her late husband. She told me, "You lose your husband, you lose your light, and you lose your house, and that's your life, isn't it?" Yet coupled with loss was also sometimes relief at the release from feeling unable to cope and from loneliness. Some residents recognised that they needed additional care support, for example when I asked Martha how she felt about leaving her home, she replied: "Listen, if you had such a hard time, you would like to get out. And I was very, very ill too." Jilly's mother had told her "I'm living too long, and I just need to be looked after, and *this* is what I want." Reverend Dawson (aged 86) had lost his wife and daughter in recent years, and he felt his grief more profoundly whilst living alone at home, describing his home as a "pretty sad place to be". He initially struggled with his move into care. I asked, "How did you settle? What made it feel a bit more like home?" He replied, "Well, several things, one was my being able to go into the kitchen and doing some cooking." This ability to engage with a personalised activity made all the difference to Reverend Dawson's well-being and ability to settle in his new care home.

Chapter summary

This chapter considered the different forms of care provision in the UK and examined some of the – often negative – perceptions of care homes. It was shown that stereotypes and associated fears surrounding loss of agency, frailty, and dependency created apprehension about moving into care which affected not only the decision-making process for adult children but also their relationship with their parents who were resistant to the move.

We considered the different types of trajectory into care, which included steep and rapid moves following a sudden health crisis in which decisions about care provision are taken out of the family's control and are taken over by health and social care professionals, as well as more gradual and uncertain journeys resulting from increasing cognitive impairment. In the latter trajectory, the decision about when to move to care was much less clear cut and in some cases caused tension within family dynamics.

Decision-making about when a parent should move into care was often made at a point in a parent's decline when the parent was no longer able to judge risk and keep themselves safe whilst living at home, or when others caring for them could no longer keep them safe. Conflict can arise between an adult child and older parent, particularly when having to challenge changing behaviours relating to dementia. However, some decisions to move were made by the older people themselves when they recognised their own limitations to coping at home.

An overarching theme throughout the transition to care surrounded the underestimation of the complexity of emotional challenges faced by both adult children and older parents, such as obligation, conflict, burden, guilt, relief, and loss. For the adult child, there is a loss of the parent they once knew, a loss of the physical presence of a parent to a home, the potential loss of a relationship with the parent and/or other family members if tensions arise, and the loss of the family home. For the older parent, there is an ongoing sense of loss and upheaval: loss of a familiar home and community, loss of independence, and a loss of purpose in having to admit that life and their care needs have changed. This, in turn, can lead to emotional responses of anger and frustration, withdrawal, or quiet acceptance and stoicism.

The negative stereotypes of care created worry amongst older adults and enormous guilt in their relatives when there was such a resistance to the move. Yet there are also some positives: there were experiences of relief once it was established that the parent had settled and was being looked after in their new home. A good care home will feel safe and there will be easier access to care when they need it. It can also be a place of connection which can be a change from the experiences of loneliness which may have preceded the move.

Looking forward, in order to better manage transitions to care, it is important that social research and policy continue to work *with* the care sector to appreciate the good work that many care homes do. It is important to continue to challenge stereotypes in the perception of care, so as to alleviate the fears associated with such a move. Other factors which can help include improving communication between homes and new residents and their families, opening homes up to the community to visit and engage with, and integrating care systems to ensure that the pre-admission phase is as smooth and as easy as possible. It is also vital that homes provide for residents according to their individual needs. The older person needs to be able to maintain a sense of identity, holding on to a part of the 'self' that they were before the move. Staff who are regularly engaged with the pre-admission process need to maintain empathy and an appreciation of how difficult this transition is for the older person and their family. And relatives who experience feelings of failure and guilt for not being able to care of their parents at home should know that even though their parent has now moved into care, this does not have to mean the end of their care contribution and involvement in their parent's life.

The next chapter explores the experience of living in care from the older parent's perspective. In particular it focuses on how meaningful attachments are made to objects associated with or involved with the transition into care – what possessions are taken into the home, who made those decisions about what to take, and which belongings help older people feel more connected to their past social identities. In particular, it is argued that clothing is central to personal and social expression. Having someone else choose your clothes for you, or having personal garments communally washed, can contribute to a sense of disconnection, not only to the social environment of the home, but also to one's sense of self (Twigg, 2013). In the transition into care most parental homes need to be sold, rented out, or returned to the council. The experience of sorting through a parent's property and clearing a home is highlighted as a particularly physical and emotionally demanding task for the adult child.

4

Materiality, clothing, and embodiment in care

Mundane, everyday objects have an important part to play in care practices and how care relationships are established and maintained. Through paying attention to how the materiality of care is constituted between bodies, objects, temporality, and space, we are able to see how objects of care can enable or constrain care practices (Buse and Twigg, 2018). There are many mundane objects which form part of an older person's world when living in care: food, personal hygiene supplies, bedding and furniture, and countless other objects which surround their daily lives. In this chapter, we will focus on objects which have a particular psychological impact upon the older person moving into care, and on the relatives and/or staff managing these objects on behalf of the older person. Most notably in the second half of the chapter we will consider the role that clothing plays in the care setting in terms of negotiating identities and mediating relationships with others.

The chapter begins by considering the personal possessions that are being transitioned from the older person's private home to the care home. It addresses the questions of how personal possessions are chosen, transported, disposed of, or managed with, or on behalf of, someone moving into care, and what impact the presence or loss of these objects has on the older person.

Possessions and 'the material convoy'

Throughout our lives we collect 'stuff': possessions that are practically useful, things that hold emotional value, and things we have not got round to using or cannot bear to throw away. At different points through the life course we may find ourselves collecting new possessions and at other points shedding them. For example, the imminent arrival of a new baby will mean buying particular items: nappies, a cot, a pram, a special teddy bear. Over time the baby will outgrow the cot, pram, and bottles and these will likely be sold, passed onto another new family, or put into storage, and there will be some items which are more immediately disposed of such as the soiled nappies. Yet the teddy may hold more sentimental attachment and may even follow the child through their entire life. Ekerdt (2018, p 30) describes this 'dynamic' and transitional 'body of belongings that accompanies people across their changing lives' as a 'material convoy'. He describes the varied reasons why we might keep items in our convoy, which then may follow us for many years, or even a lifetime. He writes,

> People keep things that are thought to be useful, have monetary value, give pleasure, symbolise oneself past and present, honour ancestors ('family things') or must be respected as gifts. People keep things because it is a virtue not to waste or trash belongings that could be used by others (Gregson, 2007), and they also keep them because they simply have the room. (Ekerdt, 2018, p 32)

Moving to care requires a significant downsizing of this 'material convoy' of possessions. There will be a lifetime of accumulated possessions which need to be sorted through and decisions need to be taken about what is kept and what is disposed of, what items are important to the older person, and what is taken with them into care. Ekerdt (2018, p 31) notes this as a particular challenge, not least because 'advancing age lays down a residue of belongings that become biographically meaningful by virtue of their duration'. There can be a sentimentality towards certain objects and when these objects are lost in the transition between living arrangements, this can create a deep sense of loss. Imagine that a teddy which has lived with a person their whole life gets lost or disposed of in the transition to care.

Material objects tell a story about the individual – who they are and 'how well life is going' (Ekerdt, 2018, p 29). In a society where the accumulation of good quality material possessions is often associated with a 'good life', when these objects are reduced to just a few simple keepsakes how must this then impact upon the way in which an older person views their life? Imagine for yourself that you had to reduce all your worldly possessions – clothing and precious objects – into one or two suitcases. What would you take? What would you leave? What would you hope happened to the items left behind? Imagine that someone else had to make those decisions for you. What do you think they would choose to represent you and your desires? Personal belongings are central to creating our sense of self and identity. Ekerdt (2018, p 38) writes that 'possessions are thus constituted by human agency, a view famously enunciated by Belk (1988), who called possessions part of the "extended self"'. Objects can represent memories, relationships, achievements, and can be invested with an emotional energy. But if someone else chooses the objects to be in your continuing, but reduced, convoy of possessions, how would they know what was important to you?

Betty (aged 86) showed me some of the personal objects she had in her care home room. Following a serious fall and subsequent hospital stay she never returned home so was unable to choose what to bring with her. She told me how her nephews selected the items she thought she might like, with her only request being a small mantle clock. I asked Betty what happened to all her other possessions? She replied with a sense of resignation and acceptance,

'Most of them went in carrier bags, and I imagine went up to charity shops. The furniture? I don't know what happened with that, went to a charity shop? And it's gone. And I haven't been back. I don't particularly want to go back, because that could upset the applecart, as I would put it, to settling in here.'

Betty's description of not wanting to 'upset the applecart' was just one example of how older people in my research restrained themselves from complaining and resigned themselves to letting go of things that perhaps might have mattered more to them than they wanted to reveal. There was a relinquishment of their own wishes and desires in order not to upset care staff or their relatives, and so not to appear too demanding. Betty went on to describe how she "didn't get a lot of say" in the possessions she brought to the home. She said, "There's little things now that I think, 'Oh, I wish I'd have got so and so'. But I haven't, and it's no good brooding on it." Sadly, her nephews did not pick out the mantle clock for her, and she also particularly missed her manicure set (something which would have enabled self-care), and her photos (her links to her past and her memories). But like many other older people she was resolute and looked for the positives, declaring "I'm spoilt. I have got some nail files here somewhere. I can't find them. I've got my perfume and I've got my pepper pot!" Ekerdt (2018, p 36) poses a question: 'Does age also shift the value and meaning of things? Perhaps different things come to matter more. Perhaps symbolic things displace useful ones, and objects that embody the past displace things that promise future pleasure or action.' This reminded me of Betty's perfume and her pepper pot: simple, mundane objects that perhaps most of us take for granted. However, in Betty's world they were vital. The scent of her perfume will create emotional associations, allowing her to relive memories of the past, and enable an expression of identity. The pepper pot too was important. Through adding pepper, she was able to gain some autonomy and control over how her food could taste. Furthermore, possessions connect to our past social identities, reminding us of a time gone by, and these memories can bring us comfort and joy. The little vintage glass pepper shaker was perhaps a link to Betty's past mealtimes with family, and its use was something that embodied her past.

Martha (aged 90) described how distant relatives cleared her home of her possessions, but they had been quite thoughtful in the items that were brought to the care home. On her wall hung a box frame containing a tiny child's pair of slippers covered in red dust. She told me the story of how, when living in Africa as a young woman, and unable to have children of her own, she cared for a child – "little Johnny" – as if he was her own for many years. Her husband had been posted to Africa in the war and she had set up a kindergarten for the army children. One mother there was expecting another child and was unable to cope. She had said to Martha that she could keep her disabled son Johnny. Martha recalled, "[the] mother said 'You can have him. You can have him'. Like that! And [my husband] said, 'Oh yes, we would like to adopt him'. We couldn't get children, you know. We tried so hard, but they just didn't come." Martha cared for Johnny for a few years until one night his parents had to leave Africa in haste to return to Germany. They collected Johnny without any notice, taking him quickly from Martha's bed whilst he was still asleep. She never saw the boy again. Johnny had left his little slippers behind covered in the red African dust. She had kept them as a memento of her little boy for the rest of her life, along with his photograph which hung proudly beside the slippers on her wall. This was a hugely precious item, representative of a child she had loved and lost. It was clear that Martha's possessions had been chosen with care. I commented that she had "lots of nice, homely bits and pieces" and that I liked Johnny's little slippers. She replied, "I must have something that belongs to me, you know, and you can't take that away from me." It became clear that in a new and unfamiliar life world, many external things have fallen outside of the older person's control and the losses associated with a move to care are tremendous. These few sentimental belongings serve the purpose of creating continuity and connection, not only to memories, but to a part of themselves that has been threatened to be lost. Johnny's little red shoes were symbolic of a story in which the child she loved so much was lost, but also of a material possession that represented being able to keep hold of a part of him. Those shoes now represented a significant part of her life narrative and were important to her as she navigated this new phase of her life.

House clearances

When a parent transitions to care, decisions need to be made about what to do with their home and property. Parental homes often need to be sold or rented out (sometimes to pay for care) and council homes may need to be returned to the local authorities. In almost all instances the house will need to be cleared of possessions, and in some cases the property may need redecorating or updating to be marketed. Sorting out of parents' affairs, particularly their home, is one of the biggest physical and emotional challenges adult children face when their parent moves to care.

Whilst Sharon's (aged 54) mother's house was on the market, she found maintaining and clearing the property particularly stressful. There had been a break-in not long after her mum had moved into the care home, and there had been a spell of bad weather which had threatened the integrity of the building. She recalls "I didn't really have any choice, it was just a burden because with these terrible winds and what if the roof lies off, you know! I needed it to remain intact so I could sell it." Sharon spent a winter clearing her mother's possessions from the property. She said:

> 'It was tough. I could never go round there by myself and do it. I tried, like I'd go round one Saturday morning, or one evening after work, but I just couldn't be there. I found it really difficult. I felt a bit scared of being there because it was a big, big house, with a park at the back of it so it was quite isolated, very quiet. And once the TV had gone it was very isolated. Every time I put my key in the door, I would be quite scared.'

She also found that the task of house clearance distracted from the relationship she needed and wanted to maintain with her mum, describing it as "obviously very time-consuming" and "all the time I was doing that I wasn't at the home with her".

There can be a deep emotional attachment to a parent's home, particularly if the older person has lived there for many years or decades, perhaps having raised their now adult children there, and for some it may have been at the very heart of the family. The memories of the family home, described by adult child relatives, were often evocative and powerful. Fred (aged 56) told me, "I can't remember what I did last Saturday, but I can still smell and taste what the house was like from 40 years ago." Coleen (aged 45) recalled how when potential buyers came to view her father's property deeply ambivalent feelings arose in her:

> 'I thought, "How dare you be eyeing up the house. This is not your house" you know, so I had to separate the childhood me, in order to be practical and think "No, this is brilliant. This is perfect. This is what you want. Someone who loves the house, Someone who's actually going to look after the house. Someone who loves it so much they want to buy it. They're not going to trash it, they're going to look after it, which is perfect". But the child in me was going, "Oooh, noooooo!"'

Coleen's response to the house viewing was interesting, signifying a return to a psychologically infantile state which is commonly experienced when faced with the loss of one's parents. It indicated a psychic tension between her need to be grown up and her defensive state of regression. Not only was Coleen saying goodbye to the home and both her parents, but also to her childhood. Sentimental items uncovered in the property clearance may further evoke a sense of loss and grief which needs to be worked through, each item bringing up memories to be processed. Coleen remembered:

'I've got big boxes of *Smash Hits*, and I didn't want to just chuck them in the bin. I'm struggling to deal with the loss of childhood in that way, and I will eventually get rid of them, but I'd just like to read them in the warmth and just go through them once again and re-live, you know the days that you don't realise that you didn't have responsibilities – happier days, more peaceful days, more blissful days. I just like to have these magazines and a few other bits and pieces down in London with me.'

These items connected Coleen to her past identity, an identity as a child and young adult with parents. They connected her to her family history, to her past, and served as a reminder of what she is now *not*.

For the older adult, a household full of a lifetime of possessions can become a burden and increasingly difficult to manage, particularly with advancing frailty. When it comes to sorting property, the task can be overwhelmingly unmanageable for the older adult or the adult child. Ekerdt (2018, p 33) suggests that 'activity to divest items from the convoy is effortful at any stage of the life course'. This is a task which often fell to relatives. Choosing which things a parent might like, choosing which items to sell, which to give to charity, which to pass on as heirlooms, which to keep; finding important paperwork, finding all the photographs – are all tasks which need to be done, but are time-consuming and need to fit in with other life commitments. The adult child may also be juggling multiple roles, including visiting their parent, childcare, holding down a job, maintaining marital relationships, negotiating sibling dynamics, managing their own deep anxiety about their own ageing and mortality, and struggling with the grief over the series of losses involved in this transitional experience.

Alison's mother's health deteriorated quickly, and she died in hospital before a care home could be arranged. Alison had lost her mum just a couple of months before our interview, and since then she had been clearing her mother's home and preparing it for sale. When I visited Alison (aged 63) to interview her in her own home she looked tearful and overwhelmed, surrounded by large boxes full of old family photographs and sentimental possessions. She said, "It's three-quarters of an hour to get there [to her mother's house]. It's been quite hard work. We've been there most weekends to sort things. We brought all the photos home, and they were in about half a dozen different places!" Now that her mother had died, there had been an expectation that this chore of emptying the property would end, but she said, "We thought, when she died, 'Oh, we're going to have weekends back to ourselves', and obviously it hasn't worked like that. I mean, every weekend, I think, practically, since Christmas, we've been there for some reason or another." Clearing a property is a difficult task which disrupts routine, daily life, and even creates changes in the adult child's own personal space. I was struck by how many boxes Alison was surrounded by and wondered about the challenges of subsuming her mother's property into her own.

For Coleen, having to commute by train to clear her father's home, running her own household, maintaining her career, and managing her dad's care home needs, without any other family support, meant that this became an overwhelming task. She found herself going to the property to clear it every weekend and even took time off work to complete the task. She found that although her dad had cleared a lot of possessions away following the death of his wife (Coleen's mother), there was still a significant amount to dispose of or move into storage. She said, "You wouldn't believe how much stuff can fit in cupboards and drawers! It's like a Tardis effect!" This six-month period of "total upheaval", as Coleen put it, was over a cold and gloomy winter. She describes the scene:

'I was sitting there; the house was freezing cold. The house was so, so, so cold, and going through all the paperwork and trying to decide what is going to be thrown, and "What do I need keep?" "What does Dad need to keep in the Care Home?" And to be brutally honest, it would have been easier if Dad had actually passed away when he'd had that fall, because you'd just clear the house, but knowing he's still alive, knowing I need to keep things for him, knowing I have the responsibility.'

She describes a duty of responsibility to get things right for her dad, and a thoughtfulness about what his needs might be.

Delving into private property, also means delving into those spaces that the older person themselves has tried to forget about or deliberately hide away. Ekerdt (2018, p 32) writes that the 'material convoy' also includes possessions which are accumulated through 'inadvertent keeping' which 'arises from the housekeeping practice of putting things away in "backstage" areas of the home (Arnold et al, 2012; Hirschman et al, 2012)'. He writes that the habit of 'replacement consumption without disposal' means that we sometimes do not want to throw things away and instead store them in the 'margins or edges of living spaces' such as in sheds or garages (Ekerdt, 2018, p 32). Clearing a home means, necessarily, probing into these forgotten spaces in the home and disposing of things that have been stored for many years. Fred described his dad's house as "untidy and disorganised" and describes finding "tins of beans that still had 3/6d on the label" and "bank statements going back to 1972!" But another consideration when clearing a property is what might be uncovered. In particular, sorting through private drawers and paperwork or even digital files may reveal difficult, surprising, or even damaging information that was previously unknown to relatives. A father (unrelated to this study) once told me that during a house clearance following the death of his daughter, that he saw things "that a father should never see". Another daughter (remaining unidentified here) told me of distasteful things found on her father's computer when clearing his digital history. Clearing possessions is a deeply personal probe into someone's life, perhaps revealing aspects of someone's life that were previously unknown, and can result in a shift in perception of that person's character.

Coleen's experience of clearing her father's property became completely overwhelming, leading to an emotional breakdown. Given that the property was in a state of disrepair, she employed the help of an estate agent friend to help manage the refurbishment. She said, "I wanted to do it properly, and I was prepared to pay for a proper painter and decorator to get the job done." But instead of contracting professional electricians and decorators, the estate agent had employed his "college-aged son-in-law" and charged her the rates of a qualified professional. On her final weekend at the house, she had planned to make it a special event. She remembers how she planned to stay the final night in the house, "I just wanted to light a few candles and just take a moment to say goodbye to the house as it was my last weekend. I wanted to make it special because I was also saying goodbye to my mum again." But sadly, this was not to be, and she recalls:

'I turned up and that house was like a bomb had gone off! All the wallpaper had been half-stripped, it was hanging in tendrils on the wall, there was rubbish everywhere, piled, on the floor, it was horrendous! And absolutely, I don't lose my temper and that was the only time in my life I've absolutely lost it, where I lost all reason. And I phoned him [the estate agent] up and I was effing and blinding down. I just said, "I can't believe you've done this. You've ripped the soul out of the house. You knew I was coming. This is my last weekend, why can't you have painted and decorated, and the proper professionals clear up after themselves after each day". What I didn't know was his son-in-law, who was absolutely shattered, he'd done a full day at college and he's trying to do it at night. I mean, the poor lad, actually he did a pretty good job under those circumstances, but not what I'd paid for, and shabby compared to a proper job. I was effing and blinding, I had the complete red mist – I can see why people go into court and say, "I lost it. It was a foolish thing to do, and I lost it", I did lose it. I absolutely did lose it. It was my final weekend in the house, and it was ruined. I was very emotional, and very tired, cold, and really close to the edge, and he pushed me over it.'

Coleen recalls the culmination of stress from all the decisions about her father's care, the poor condition of the house, the loss of the memories, and the added stress of a family argument meant that she collapsed alone in a frightening panic attack. She describes how she felt following that phone call to the estate agent:

'I couldn't breathe, and I was on my hands and knees trying to catch my breath, and that was quite frightening. I was crying, and then crying then becomes sort of sobbing. You can say, "Nothing wrong with crying at all", but actually I'm in control, and it's only when things really get on top of you, and that did. I mean it's the only time in my life when it wasn't crying, it was like [in breath] and then suddenly you can't breathe. Everything seems to seize up and you can't breathe. And I suddenly thought, "Oh, this isn't good!" It just really shocked me. And that's when I had my moment, my breakdown. And then you get practical, and you think "No you need to breathe, because if you don't breathe then you will pass away surrounded by all this crap, so just sort yourself out and get it back together again".'

The experience was deeply distressing and overwhelming. Not only was Coleen losing her dad to a care home and grieving his eventual death, but she was also grieving her mum for a second time as if her mum's spirit had also lived within that home. She was also grieving for the house they all lived in and the possessions that had surrounded them, and she was also grieving the loss of her own sense of being a child and never being able to return to that position ever again.

Loss was a dominant emotion when managing the distribution and clearance of 'the material convoy' in the older person's home. Reverend Dawson (aged 86) had lived in his private home for over 50 years with his wife and had raised a family there. In the rush to collect possessions to take with him to the home, he found himself in ownership of things that he did not want or need, and his more precious items were lost. On a practical note, he had lost his hymn books and he needed them to write an upcoming service, but more poignantly he had lost a booklet that he had created for his late daughter, who had died aged 40. His sons took all his main furniture to a local charity shop, and some was distributed to friends. He was most upset by items that were simply taken to the local refuse centre. He told me:

'I'm afraid an awful lot was thrown away and put into a tip, and it distressed me. We had, I had an everyday China set, you know, a dinner service and tea service, which I'd used for a long, long time, and they were okay actually, and they were in a cupboard, and I said to [my son] "Look, can you wrap them up and take them to the Hospice Shop". They didn't. They threw it all in the tip because they said it was too much of a job to do.'

Ekerdt (2018) described that there was often a 'generational disconnect about household items associated with fine dining, such as china and silver sets, which the older generation prizes but the children do not want, thus complicating the transfer of these things within the family (Ekerdt et al, 2012)' (Ekerdt, 2018, p 37). Items such as a special china set have often stayed with a family for many years or even decades, representing a sense of continuity, with treasured memories of their use, and are often treated with great care, so for Reverend Dawson to see such items devalued and carelessly disposed of was particularly distressing.

Clothing

Clothing is a particular type of possession invested with personal and social expression, and embodied personhood (Buse and Twigg, 2014). In her studies of dementia and dress, Twigg (2010, p 223) noted that clothes represent the 'environment closest in'. She writes that the closeness of the cloth to the skin is important for the person living with dementia in that it gives them a 'sensory grasp of surroundings' which is often 'strange', 'reduced or confused'. It is the feel of the fabric which can bring the wearer a sense of 'security and comfort' and 'reassurance' (Twigg, 2018, pp 189–90). She further recognised that clothing had the ability to allow a presentation of self, as the person they once were.

How someone dresses offers an important signal to others in maintaining a particular identity. Clothing is an expression of selfhood, and it can be disconcerting if relatives see their parents in the 'wrong' clothes, or if they are found wearing something that their parent would never normally wear if they had a choice. Care home organisations often have communal systems for washing clothing and bedding. These large loads of boiled washes can dictate what clothes can be washed in the care home. Certain fabric types are damaged by the washes, and clothing often goes astray in the distribution of the cleaned items. Ward et al (2014) note that this means that appearances are 'shaped both by the social and material environment, eroding the choice and agency of the individual'. Joan (aged 87) told me that her daughter pops in every other day to see her and she will now take her washing home with her. Joan complained about the washing system and how her new items had been damaged in the process: "I had nice new bras when I came here, and they got absolutely ruined in the laundry here – all the hooks are bent and broken – and it's such a shame." Valentina (aged around 90 years old), too, had temporarily lost some items – a nightdress and some socks. She recalled that they came back to her after a few weeks of "probably being in somebody else's room". She said it was a bit "off-putting" because "you don't know whether they've been worn or not". Sharon (aged 54) told me how she labelled all her mother's clothes when she moved into care, but they still got mixed up in the laundry. She said:

'They tend to get mixed up a bit, and at first I was sort of, not angry – I don't get angry – but, you know, just disturbed by it, but now I just think, "There's nothing I can do about it. They're clean. They're coming back from the laundry", so she sometimes has other people's clothes on, and that's a bit weird, but you just kind of accept that she doesn't recognise her own clothing.'

It can be unsettling to see a parent dressed differently to how they would ordinarily dress. Identity can become easily transgressed when clothes are picked out for the older person or become muddled and distributed incorrectly by the laundry system. For staff, deciding on what clothes an older person might want to wear may appear a simple care task and arguably it is one that is not taken account of enough in care homes policies. It is often a task which is subsumed into the 'daily task-oriented, time-pressured routines of care provision' (Ward et al, 2014, p 64). But for older residents, having someone else choose your clothes, or having personal garments communally washed and distributed once in the home, can contribute to a sense of disconnection, not only to the social environment of the home, but also to a sense of self and others.

The volunteers I interviewed in the care homes sometimes noticed that residents would occasionally be dressed without thought or care for how they would look. Lydia, a volunteer, told me how she had felt angry when she saw a female resident dressed in a pink shirt and orange cardigan and she, along with the resident herself, didn't think that it was a good match. Lydia complained to me, "Why does someone else get to say what she is wearing?" Adult child relative Jilly (aged 68) was more understanding about her mother's state of dress and associated this with part of her mother's cognitive deterioration rather than the fault of the care staff. She told me that her mother has now become unable to choose her own clothes or dress herself. She said:

'They [the carers] choose what she's going to wear, and I keep suggesting to her that she should look in her wardrobe and pick out – like the trousers she's got on now, or a dress – and she says she knows she should. And so sometimes she says they choose things which are not very appropriate, or that she would never have chosen. But they're hanging in her wardrobe after all, so it's not their fault! But if she can't quite sort of say just exactly what she wants, I'm afraid that's her problem, to be honest.'

Like many other possessions from the 'material convoy', the choice of clothing to bring to the home was also often mediated by a relative, inevitably determining what was available for the older person to wear. Mildred (aged 86) described how her daughter-in-law had chosen the clothes to take to the home. She recalled: "[My daughter-in-law] decided and brought me in the clothes that I want – well, she *thinks* I would want, let's put it that way! – had a good clear out, in other words! And that's it." Similarly, 86-year-old Betty's nephews chose what possessions she should take to the home and picked out the clothes she would keep. She said, "I've got clothes, some of them I might have brought, some of them I might not have done. They weren't my choice, some of them, although they were my choice originally, I might not have brought them here with me." Imagine, just for a moment, if someone was to go through your wardrobe on your behalf and pick out clothes for you to wear. What might they choose and what would you think about those choices?

There is an interconnection between the subjective and lived body experience (embodiment) and the way the body is constructed. Clothing is central to the construction and 'the presentation of self in everyday life' (Goffman, 1959). When this performance of self is disrupted by the older person or is not upheld and maintained correctly by those caring for them, this can create a cause for concern amongst the adult child relatives. In her study, Whitaker (2009, p 165) found that visiting family members would 'search for physical/bodily traces and signs' on their older relative's body in order to 'make observations of care given or neglected by staff and interpret and try to understand the state of health of the old one'. She terms this as an 'archaeology of kinship care' describing how 'every visit is a reminder of the family's absence and of the period of time that has passed since the last visit, and every new visit requires a "time, space, and body analysis", based on available traces and signs' (Whitaker, 2009, p 165). This was described by care staff as part of a focus group in my studies too. A staff member described a female resident who had always liked to apply her makeup and "look really presentable", but it was "getting to a stage where she was forgetting to do that". The staff would try to remind her to apply her makeup as usual, but one day she said to them "I don't want that anymore". The staff member in the group recalled how:

'She was changing, and her family found that really, really hard to accept. They wanted their mother to put her makeup on still, and they wanted their mother to be the way she had always been, all the time. And they found that really hard to accept, that that wasn't her anymore. That was hard.'

Care staff, in the focus group, described how the resident became progressively worse, eventually moving to a specialised unit. They described how they had to have several meetings with the resident's family and keep a chart about how their mum was feeling through the week and whether she had wanted her makeup on each day: "We would basically keep a record of things and record everything so families could see what she was like on a day-to-day basis, so they could just get a good idea of how they were changing really." In this given example, the resident's body was 'a primary tool for interpretation' (Whitaker, 2009, p 165). The visiting relative may view the body of the older person as something to be physiologically surveilled and monitored for signs of change, whether positive or negative, acceptable or not acceptable. I recognised that amongst the adult children and amongst the visiting volunteers there was the significant 'noticing' that goes on during a care home visit, looking for clues on the site of the older person's body and within their immediate environment which might offer any indications of change in the person and/or their quality of care.

Chapter summary

The materiality of care draws attention to the mundane objects of care and the role they play in the life worlds of those who interact with them. Ekerdt (2018, p 29) writes:

> The life course is commonly charted by intangibles, as a progression of roles, statuses, relationships, emotions, identities and levels of well-being. Yet the life course also has a physical, material reality: it is enacted and embodied with things, it proceeds in the service of things, and the passage of time propels people towards the consumption of things.

Material objects, particularly clothing, play a central role in the embodiment of ageing and care. The interaction between objects and the lived experience of the body enables identities to be constructed and past identities to be re-enacted. Objects become a biographical resource telling stories about the past, reigniting memories, and creating a sense of comfort or reassurance in navigating the transition to care. Objects can enable autonomy and control, even on the smallest of scales such as filing one's own nails or flavouring a meal with pepper.

The material convoy is a fluid, dynamic body of possessions which travels with the person through the whole of their life course – amassing and shedding items at different moments in time. But possessions can also be a burden: things that have been hidden away, things that have been forgotten about, and items that have accumulated layers of sentimentality can all be difficult to manage and dispose of, particularly when struggling with the challenges of advancing age and frailty. The transition to care involves significant moments in the disposal of the majority of this convoy and downsizing to just the smallest collection of items, often selected by someone else. Sadly, this reflects the often-paternalistic way in which some older people are treated, with actions done unto them, and with little say in their preferences and wishes even when they have capacity to have a say in such important decisions.

This chapter is a call to whoever is clearing a property to carefully consider the objects that are meaningful to the older person and to have 'caring conversations' (Dewar and Nolan, 2013) about what the older person wants. The same is true for clothing; how the older person adorns their body with clothing and accessories plays a central role in how they express their identity, both an identity which preceded care home life and their identity now in this new environment. When this element of choice is reduced or removed this can have important consequences for the ways in which the older person can enable their identity, maintain a connection with their past, experience a sense of safety and comfort, and, moreover, mediate their relationships with others.

The following chapter continues with the challenges faced by older people as they settle into their new care home, and how they find new avenues of self-expression, autonomy, and friendship. It highlights the relationships that are made in the home between the older person and other residents, staff, and visiting relatives.

5

Social connections and relationship building in residential care

Creating and maintaining good social connections and relationships when transitioning to a care home are central to promoting good physical and mental health of older people and to maintaining a good quality of life. Older people relate to others within a complex web of social networks which situates them in relationships with other residents, relatives, visitors, external health-care professionals, and internal care and ancillary staff in their care home. If this social network of connections is operating successfully, then it can offer emotional support, physical care, social engagement, and a sense of belonging. Williamson (2010) outlines a number of key indicators relating to the quality of life for older people, which include healthy relationships with others and having someone to talk to, a comfortable living environment, good physical health, a sense of humour, independence, the ability to communicate, a sense of personal identity, the ability and opportunity to engage in activities, and the ability to practise faith or religion. Nolan et al's (2006) 'Senses Framework' lists a sense of security, a sense of belonging, a sense of community, a sense of purpose, a sense of achievement, and a sense of significance as the elements required for a good quality of life in a care home for the residents, but also for the good quality working environment for the staff and a good environment for visiting. My Home Life England (2022a) sets out a framework for achieving good relationships and quality of life for all that live, die, visit, and work in care home settings. It writes that, 'We need to consider what gives each individual a sense of security (feel safe), belonging (feel part of things), continuity (make connections between past, present and future), purpose (have goals), achievement (moving towards their goals) and significance (matter as a person)' (My Home Life England, 2022b).

This chapter explores how older people and their visiting adult child relatives enable an expression of these well-being indicators when they transition to long-term care. How do adult child relatives and the care staff create a comfortable and welcoming environment for the older person in the care facility, and what is important in this process? How can older people discover a sense of autonomy, independence, and identity expression through these relationships? And how can communication be facilitated in the care environment when there are limits to physical mobility and cognition?

Connections with other residents

Imagine for a moment that you are an older person moving into an unfamiliar space with people you do not know and perhaps would not choose to be with. How might that feel? Imagine that you cannot hear or see very well. How might that hinder the relationships you are able to build? Imagine that you make a new friend in the home, only for them to forget you the next day.

One set of key quality-of-life indicators outlined by Williamson (2010) is grouped around older people's relationships with other people, and one of the most significant network of relationships is with the other residents living in care. My research found that despite care home residents often being surrounded by plenty of other people, many still felt terribly lonely. There were environmental restrictions which inhibited relationship building between residents. Many older people were using mobility devices to support functional mobility and struggled to navigate their physical environment without support or without a fear of falling. This, and the separation by individual wing-backed chairs arranged side-by-side in the lounges, meant that many older people were left unable to easily communicate with one another. The immovability (and often territoriality) of the heavy armchairs meant that seating could not be easily rearranged to sit and talk with someone new.

When talking with residents, I had to get close to the ear or face of a resident to hear what they were saying. There were frequent breaks in conversation because someone could not hear or could not remember what has been said, which led to conversations between residents spiralling in different directions. One resident, Jackie (aged approximately in her mid 80s), had a very quiet, soft voice and was unable to make herself heard by other residents. She was physically disabled with her head bent low into her chest, and unable to lift it to project her voice. This inability to move her head or be heard meant that this resident was becoming increasingly lonely. She told me despondently, "I don't talk to anyone. I keep myself to myself. If I had a fish in a bag and it could talk, I would talk back to it."

Often residents got frustrated with one another and were sometimes unable to comprehend why a fellow resident might not remember a conversation. Most residents suffered some degree of dementia or deafness or a combination of the two, which made fluid and intelligent conversation difficult. Resident, Rita (aged approximately in her mid 80s) said, "several of the people here, well I shouldn't say this, but they are a bit you know, well there is one lady I sit next to, she is ever so nice, but she can't remember what happens ten minutes before", and resident Maeve (aged 79) said, "I can't talk to some of them because they're deaf". Conversations at mealtimes were particularly difficult due to the acoustics of the dining room; the clattering of plates meant that the residents were unable to hear each other at the table, so instead sat and ate in silence.

Upon entering care, perhaps the only thing that residents have in common is their agedness and frailty, and perhaps in times gone by they may never have chosen to been friends with one another. They may have little in common and find it difficult to socialise when there is little to discuss. When I asked Betty (aged 86) if she had made friends in the home, she replied, "Not as such. I talk to them, but like everybody else, we do nothing but sleep!" Reverend Dawson (aged 86) described how some other residents "drove him round the bend" and that he had "nothing in common with anybody there" and that he finds relating to others in the home "very, very difficult". However, he had recently made three friends in the home, and they sit together for mealtimes now. He said, "We're a little trio. We talk the same language."

However, there were also moments of connection between residents. On occasions I saw small groupings of residents, usually women, sat together at a table enjoying tea and conversation together. It was noticeable that talk was more easily facilitated around a table, than having to peer around their armchairs. There were small moments of compassion and care between residents too. As I sat next to Dot (aged in her 80s) in the lounge, another lady got up and complained loudly "I am getting more and more bored", to which Dot replied, "Don't worry I will cheer you up!" I also noticed on another visit a female resident talking to the lady sat next to her. The first woman asked her neighbour kindly if she was warm enough. The second woman replied that she was "OK", because she had "this nice, knitted, cardigan" which she had "put over her lap". She continued by saying that it was "a lovely cardigan" and that "the knit was quite unusual". The first lady replied, "it is unusual, just like me" and they laughed quietly together. The first woman explained to me that she had lent her the cardigan because "she said she was cold, so I said to put it round her". These were small moments of social connection and compassion with residents attending to each other's needs. The cardigan was an object of clothing which had a mediating effect on the relationships with others; in this case opening up communication and interactions between lounge-room neighbours.

I wondered then how these residents must feel when their care home friend that they have being looking out for, or who looks out for them, goes into hospital, takes permanently to their bed, or even dies. Care home friendships felt underestimated in their impact on the emotional well-being of care home residents. This was most acutely noticed in some care homes which did not find it necessary to inform (or 'did not want to upset') the residents when a member of their community died. It was certainly noted as good practice when at least a photo, a candle, or a memorial booklet was laid out in a public space, such as a hallway, when a resident had died.

Intimacy and sexuality

Just as the arrangement of wing-backed chairs precluded communication in the lounges, I noticed that physical layout of a care home plays an important role in the relationships that are allowed to develop in that space. Single beds in bedrooms prohibit intimate relationships and form part of a continuing exclusion from sexual citizenship in later life. Older people's bodies in care homes are only generally touched through the caring context, by care staff providing intimate but instrumental and practical care support. The body is no longer treated as a site of pleasure, love, and/or eroticism, and sexual connections are often dismissed, ridiculed, or made secretive. Developing romantic connections between residents were frequently infantilised and seen as 'silly'.

This experience of exclusion from intimacy was starkly highlighted when interviewing care home resident Jessie (aged approximately in her mid 80s) and her husband who was visiting with a young female volunteer in attendance. Jessie was physically very disabled, unable to move any part of her body apart from her face and fingers. She was very dependent upon carers for her physical welfare. Cognitively she was well, but she was quite depressed. She told me with tears in her eyes, "Oh I would give anything to go home." She had been married for 63 years, and although her husband visited her for eight hours every single day, he was unable to stay the night. She said, "We have always had a lot of love for each other. I am only just sorry that I am not able to do all the things I would love to do." Her husband told me that the day before that they had a "really good laugh" when two carers were putting Jessie into a hoist, and she had declared loudly "take me up to bed, I am going to make love now!" As he told me this story, he laughed loudly and so did the volunteer. I smiled weakly in response but then noticed Jessie's face had dropped. She was deadly serious; this was something she really desired. She wanted to be taken seriously about her need for intimacy and touch. Not necessarily sex, but to lie in bed with her husband as she had done for decades before. She said, "It is about going to bed with him to be quite honest. I truly miss it." She turned to me and said, "I am glad *you* take me seriously." There was so much love between the couple and Jessie was desperately longing for that connection with her husband. It was about her human need to be intimate and was an essential part of her relationship that I felt was being denied to her. There were double rooms in some of the care homes and there was, when available, the opportunity for couples to join the care home together. However, when one spouse was in a care home and the other remained at the family home, there was little space for them to spend intimate time together. And there was very little opportunity for new relationships to form into anything more than a friendly hello in the lounge.

Connections with staff

Care staff work under enormous physical, psychological, and time pressure, often leaving them feeling over-burdened. This has been exacerbated by staffing shortages across the care sector, and this situation has worsened as a result of the COVID-19 pandemic (Lightfoot and Moone, 2020). Staff carry out a range of instrumental care tasks such as personal care, assisting with mobility, providing meals, and cleaning spaces, and although these are carried out with care, we found that in some homes that there was much less time for social and emotional connection with residents.

On one particular occasion my colleague Chris Tanner and I were observing life in the home simultaneously. I was shadowing a volunteer, Ashleigh, and Chris was shadowing a care home staff member. Whilst there, an entertainer came to perform for the residents. My field notes captured the following scene:

> The entertainer sang old-fashioned songs with actions to a lounge full of residents. Some were asleep but most seemed to be enjoying it. The two activities leaders were dancing and encouraging the residents to dance along with them. There was one lady who was very enthusiastic, dancing in her chair and singing along. Another man, opposite the doorway where Ashleigh and I were standing was beckoning us in. We were pretending to dance half-heartedly in the doorway. I wanted to join in a bit more and I think if I had been a volunteer myself I might have gone up to a resident and joined in with them, rather than hiding in a doorway. I felt guilty about not doing anything and just standing there watching whilst Chris was running around after the staff member who he was observing. The staff member was hurriedly grabbing a hoist and attending to a resident in the conservatory. Chris seemed extremely busy chasing after the staff member (he was even running on occasion!), whereas I felt like I was a bit redundant and a bit on the side lines, not knowing what I was supposed to be doing. I wondered how much of that Ashleigh feels herself, about not knowing quite what we are meant to be doing. It was fun, and I was enjoying myself, but I did think, 'am I supposed to be enjoying myself?'

What was notable in this observation was that the pace of activity was starkly different between the staff members who were attending to physical care tasks, compared to the volunteers who were assigned to keep residents company and entertain them. Following this observation Chris and I interviewed the manager of the home. She said, "The staff feel a lot of guilt about sitting down and talking to a resident" and "We need to change that culture. Those five minutes of intimacy are very important but if they sit down they think they are being lazy." This I think was reflected by the enormous guilt I felt in getting involved in the intimate, socially connecting work with residents – the feeling of 'not working' and 'enjoying myself', rather than being more involved in the demanding instrumental care tasks that Chris was shadowing. My Home Life's 'Focusing on Relationships' framework distinguishes the experiences of 'safety', 'belonging', 'purpose', 'achievement', 'continuity', and 'significance' as being central to developing relationships in a care home. It is therefore critical that staff are empowered and enabled to take the time to build social connections between staff and residents without feeling 'guilty' or 'lazy'. There needs to be recognition that quality care is more than the instrumental, physical tasks, but also involves relationality, empathy, and connecting. It may also be valuable to reflect upon 'what is being avoided amongst such busy-ness?'

Another striking feature of the social relationships that older people had in care (across the whole social network) was the temporary nature of the connections. I found staff were often very busy and their conversations with residents were fleeting or happened during an attendance to the older person's intimate care needs, such as whilst taking them to the toilet, bathing them, dressing them, or putting them in bed. Visitors to the home did not usually stay very long, and there was sometimes little to do or talk about. Connections formed by staff, visitors, and volunteers with older people could also be temporary due to their being forgotten from one visit to the next, residents moving care facilities, or even dying. Volunteers faced the challenge of building a relationship with an older person on one visit, only for it to be completely forgotten by the next. This was initially quite painful and disheartening for some volunteers and one of the programme volunteers resigned as a result. The challenge in these relationships is to help staff and visitors to recognise the immediate value of their connection, even if it is to be shortly forgotten.

Care staff regularly manage vulnerability, pain, and distress in their work role whilst being expected to simultaneously offer up positive actions and feelings. They had to be able to accommodate and contain this contradiction without disengaging, practically and emotionally, from those that they cared for. Staff and volunteers were regularly faced by the loss of people they had developed friendships with, having invested time and energy into that relationship. On one particular occasion, a volunteer had developed a strong bond with a particular resident and paid them a regular visit, only to find a new resident in their room. She recalled, "[The staff] don't tell me, for example, if somebody's died, and that's quite hard. I find it really, really quite difficult when people die because I get very fond of them, and then, it almost …, somebody else is in their room, and I find that really hard." Sadly, we noticed that volunteers and visitors were not always informed of the death of a resident because they were not afforded the same communication privileges as staff.

By virtue of being in care, residents are in a position of vulnerability, and they are moving into a place where their behaviour can be restricted either by other people or by the limits of their own mobility. We found that residents did not want to complain about their care because they had a fear of upsetting those who cared for them. One volunteer said, "[the residents] don't want to make waves". One resident we observed speaking to a manager asked, "If I tell you something you won't be upset will you and you won't make me move?" Adult child relative Jilly (aged 68) said that her mum "doesn't like complaining and she won't let me. When I complain, I don't tell her, because she'll be furious if she knows I've gone to someone. She thinks they'll take it out on her." From the older person's perspective, the worst thing for them was to upset the rhythm, stability, and routine of daily life in their care home, which kept them feeling safe. However, reticence to complain does not lead to improvements in care. Instead, feedback and challenges should be welcomed and even actively encouraged in care settings in order to create a culture of transparency. This would help to empower residents in the expression of their needs, and enable staff to be trained in recognising, understanding, and attending to those needs.

Intimate personal care

Personal care can include support with a range of care tasks such as bathing, cleansing or creaming the skin, shaving, oral hygiene, helping someone to the toilet, washing intimate areas of the body, or changing catheters or stoma bags. Intimate personal care can change the nature and quality of the relationship between two people, particularly as the care receiver is in a position of ultimate vulnerability. It is important in these caregiving situations that the older person is empowered to carry out as much of their own care as they are able to and can express their likes and dislikes and what they are comfortable with. However, in positions where they have to receive intimate care, it should be delivered with dignity, safety, empathy, competence, compassion, and privacy. This form of caregiving has the potential to position the older person in a state of lesser power, and the experience of touch may feel embarrassing, frustrating, or even frightening and assaulting, particularly when the care receiver has advanced dementia and has forgotten the experience of being washed or touched. Woodspring (2016, p 86) writes that:

Repeatedly, Twigg refers to 'real bodies,' taking the mundane experience of those in care and, in particular, being bathed, out of the theoretical realm and into the real world of being touched and handled by care staff. It is this materiality that drives the reader to a sense of tangible ageing corporeality in care.

This quotation highlights the experience of touching and being touched in embodied care giving. Imagine for yourself, how it might be to receive such intimate care from someone else. Perhaps they are a new and unfamiliar member of staff. Perhaps they are a staff member who you have forgotten about, but who has cared for you before. Perhaps they are a staff member you do not like or trust. The delivery of the care in these relationships has the potential to be particularly disconcerting and uncomfortable. However, when such care is delivered well in a trusting way, there is the potential for intimate care to facilitate good and close social connections.

Adult child relatives may also want to deliver personal care to their parents, and this can be an important way of building and maintaining their relationships with parents. This may take the form of bathing a parent, helping to dress them, or even becoming involved in more intimate cleaning. However, they are more likely to become involved in acts of 'lighter bodily care' (Whitaker, 2009, p 162), comprising tasks such as brushing hair, applying face cream, or painting and filing fingernails. These small care acts not only help the older person look or feel nice, but they also make the relatives feel useful and more involved, make visits feel more rewarding, and are a way of building platonic intimacy. In my research, it was found that the care home managers were quite aware of the need to make relatives feel confident in engaging in these acts of care service. One manager said:

'Some of them will feel that they're handing over their relative, and that they can't help any more. One of the things we try and do is say, "No! If you've been doing these things for your parent for …" – however long that might be – "if you still want to do some of those things you can. We're just here to do the things that you don't feel able to do any more" but "even if you want to still wash your mother, or bath your father, we are not going to stop you doing that".'

The manager, Tina, said that relatives needed to be "open-minded" about the care they can continue to offer to their parents. She said that, "If someone said 'I would really like to give my mum a bath, is there a way we can arrange a time?'" then that was something they could plan and facilitate. Tina also recognised the importance of care home residents building relationships with other people who did not attend to their personal, intimate care needs. She acknowledged that even though the carers were extremely good at "building and sustaining positive relationships" with the residents they cared for, it was also "really important for people to have diverse relationships and also to have relationships with people who do not see them undressed". She went on to say that she could think of only three people amongst the staff who would not have seen a resident in a state of undress or in the bath or shower.

Autonomy and activity

One of the principal ways of connecting with staff and other residents on a social level in a care home is through the involvement in the home's activities. However, with a large group of people of varying abilities and coming from a range of backgrounds – all with their unique skills and interests – it is difficult to engage a large group in activities which will suit everyone. Activities staff had to balance the physical abilities of the residents with the provision of meaningful activities for them. One manager said, "With activities you're trying to appease so many people with so many different expectations and interests."

My colleague Chris Tanner and I observed life in the care homes and the activities of community visitors. We found that community visitor volunteers were instrumental in arranging for a range of group activities for residents, including bringing in reminiscence boxes from the local museum, campaigning successfully for funding for iPads for residents, setting up a Scrabble club, and arranging future outings. Well-run and thought-through activities fostered greater companionship between residents, improved social engagement with the local community, and greater feelings of well-being and resilience. What was evident was the need for care homes to recognise the individuality of residents and to offer opportunity for personal growth and development, rather than viewing care home residents as passive receivers of entertainment.

Residents welcomed the opportunity to play a useful, active role within the home, instead of being on the receiving end of care. Residents engaged in activities which increased their sense of autonomy and independence had higher levels of satisfaction with life in care. Betty (aged 86) liked to help the activities coordinator to set up activities three times a week. Mildred (aged 86) had high praise for her activities coordinator, saying, "There's a lot of entertainment goes on … they all do something to involve everybody, which is nice – there's nobody left out. It's very, very, as I say co-ordinated, well organised." All of the care homes I observed had visiting groups from the local community. Daisy (aged 90) said about the visiting students from the sixth form college, "I find them interesting, more than anything. See what's going on in the outer world." Another home had visits from children from a local primary school who had come and sung Christmas carols to the residents. Joan (aged 87) had taken part, and said, "Oh it's lovely to see them" and she described how "it makes you feel you can open your eyes wider and take it all in". My Home Life England (2023) runs an 'intergenerational linking' project and advocates for the advantages of such connections. It notes that:

By giving those taking part the opportunity to come together to share in new experiences, learning, stories and laughter, particularly individuals that otherwise may never meet, we're striving to create meaningful intergenerational friendships that are mutually beneficial, strengthen community connection and deepen understanding of each other and how we all live together. Over time, we hope that long-term, sustainable links will develop between the participating schools, youth groups and care homes. (My Home Life England, 2022)

Music is also extremely important and evocative as an activity in care settings, offering a powerful connection to shared experiences and relationships, and helping to stimulate memories, particularly with residents living with advanced dementia. On one visit I saw the care home's activities coordinator entertaining the lounge of twelve residents with a karaoke of old-time tunes, with the television screen displaying the lyrics. He was encouraging the residents to join in with the sing-along, offering them a remote control as a makeshift microphone. One woman aged 103 appeared to be asleep through most of the singing but as soon as 'Baby Face' came on, her face lit up and she started to sing along, and even when she looked like she was asleep again, her slippered-foot was still gently tapping.

The NICE guidelines recommend that older people in care homes should be 'offered opportunities during their day to participate in meaningful activity that promotes their health and mental wellbeing' (Care Quality Statement 1). The guidelines ask care homes to encourage residents to become more involved in their activities of their own daily life, and 'meaningful activity' can include simply encouraging a resident to be involved in routine personal care tasks (NICE, 2019). Care services should help to ensure that older people retain autonomy as far as possible, even in these small acts of self-care in everyday life. If the care organisation holds strict temporal control over the home and the residents' lives, this can feel depersonalising and institutionalising. Most residents valued having control over the little things in their day-to-day lives, like engaging in good company and conversation, and being involved in meaningful and personalised activities.

In particular, residents valued having a say over when they went to bed, and in some homes, relative freedom over when and what they ate. Dot (aged approximately in her 80s) said cheerfully:

'From what I hear of other homes compared to this one, it knocks spots off the others, it really does. I tell them what we do and what we get, and they are like "we don't get that!" We can go to bed when we like can't we? We can practically do what we like.'

Another female resident sat in the lounge announced loudly, "I am going to stay up all night!" The manager replied, "OK, Jean, but why do you want to do that?" Jean declared, "Cos I want to stay up all night." Later the manager told me that

> 'Residents go to bed when they want and if Jean wants to stay up all night then she can. She might well go to bed at 3am, but as long as she knows that at 1pm they will put the hoover round the lounge, that's OK. If that's what she would do in her own home then that's what she can do here.'

It was important for older people to feel comfortable in their routines and for these to be as similar as possible to those they were used to at home.

Many of the residents I spoke to did not want to get involved in communal activities in their home and I wondered about the drive towards 'activity' and 'doing' that was being impressed upon older people by the younger generations of care staff, volunteers, and visitors. One manager said, for example, that it was "difficult to engage older people though activities" as "there's not the get up and go". But I reflected upon this and wondered why there needed to be a 'get up and go'. Some of the older voices of dissent regarding group activities were tired and wanted peace and quiet away from the hustle and bustle. Mr Randall (aged 98) told me, "As you get older you don't want to do more." I witnessed one volunteer ask a lounge of residents "Is there anything you want to do?" and an older lady replied, "When you get to this age you have had enough". Some residents found it physically too much of a chore to leave their rooms. Joan (aged 87) was very physically disabled, had to use a hoist and an extra-large wheelchair which was hard for staff to get through doorways, and had to take oxygen cylinders wherever she went. It felt like too much of a physical effort for Joan to move and she felt like it was a burden to request assistance. She described her typical day to me, "I sit in here all morning, and I go to bed in the afternoon. I stay in bed till the morning. I don't get up again." Similarly, Missy (aged 90) had a bad hip that meant she had to use a walking frame, which she had decorated with fairy-lights. She had been quite interested in what group activity was going on downstairs, but she was worried that if she did not like it or needed the toilet during the activity then it would take her a very long time to walk back to her room. She said, "When you're old. I mean, I'm 90! It gives me all I can do to get up and walk with this."

The little things

The most common complaints I witnessed in care homes concerned 'the little things' that could have been easily sorted out, and when these little things went unaddressed, anxieties were quickly raised. One manager said "It is the small things that are so important to the quality of care. Things like having your tea made right. Residents often don't like to say anything so little things like that often go unnoticed."

I witnessed a litany of 'little things' that the volunteers and visiting relatives helped residents with which helped smooth the course of their day. This included posting cards and letters, reading the paper to a resident, doing up the zip on a handbag which had got stuck, asking the staff for some grapes. It was the ability (and time) to notice which was key. Residents could be easily become upset by things that were easily remedied by a short conversation or action such as moving the flowers, making a tea instead of a coffee, having an address read out to them on a letter, letting them know the day of the week, making sure a bell was pressed and a staff member coming quickly, holding a hand, or passing a tissue. On one visit a resident looked quite sad and the volunteer asked what was wrong. The female resident replied that she had had an upsetting letter informing her of the death of someone she knew but she couldn't read who it was and who had written the letter. The volunteer read the letter and address out loud to her, and although the news was indeed sad, it was not the death of the person she initially thought it was and having that disconfirmed reassured the resident.

One volunteer said that attending to these small tasks helped stop "silly things happening within the home". She said that because staff were so busy "they don't always see little things that are happening" but that it was the little things that were really important for the residents. Mr Randall (aged 98) found that the little things were frequently missed, and this annoyed him intensely. He told me that at mealtimes there would be three or four of them sat at the table in the dining room, but rarely was the table laid for them all and he would frequently be without cutlery. He said "They bring you in your porridge. I said, 'Oh, do I eat it with my hands?' I said, 'I haven't got a spoon'." He said that his friend would take one from another table, but he would tell him off and say " 'No, put that back, that's stealing'". But if he asked care staff for a spoon, they would get distracted by other tasks and he would sit there and "by the time they get in with the spoon, your porridge is cold" and he would send it back to the kitchen. He then feared that he would be moaned about, and staff would say " 'Oh, he's always got a problem!'" These small, seemingly inconsequential things can have a big impact on the mental well-being of residents and the degree to which they feel cared and thought about.

I found that volunteers and visitors had a greater ability – and more time – to 'notice' things which may have been lost in the busyness of the care home system. Aside from being too busy to notice, another reason why little things got overlooked was that these tasks seemed to go unrecognised and underappreciated within the workplace environment. Addressing micro-issues in a home was not necessarily something tangible which would be recognised and praised by management. Yet we noticed that it was through the little things that bigger, more serious issues were addressed. For instance, one resident was afraid to go to the dentist and a volunteer finally persuaded her to attend her appointment, offering to accompany her. This appointment led to the identification of a much more serious underlying diagnosis of terminal lung cancer for the resident. Without this 'noticing' by the volunteer, this condition may have been missed. As a result of this experience, the volunteer developed a very close bond with the resident and sat with her on every visit until the resident's death a few months later.

I found in my observations, that this capacity to 'notice' was a fragile ability. Visitors to the home saw things differently to the staff, often from a new and sometimes divergent perspective. The bodies of care home residents may be viewed by care staff through a lens of instrumental care provision – tasks that need to be completed within a shift. The perspective of a visitor can see things that perhaps have been taken for granted by staff who spend extended periods of time in the home. And a visiting adult child relative will likely view their older parent with an intimate personal lens which remembers their previous autonomous, independent identity invested with all their history, stories, relationships, hopes, and dreams.

Connections between adult child relatives and their older parents

The relationship between the adult child and their older parent shifts with the transition to care. Adult children often feel intensely guilty about the move, and this can impact upon the way they relate to their parent and to the care staff. For an adult child, visiting a parent living in care can be challenging on a practical level if they do not live locally, and visits can feel disappointing and pointless if a parent with dementia forgets them. This section of the chapter focuses on some of these challenges.

Guilt and the impact on social connections

Miceli and Castelfranchi (2018, p 710) define guilt as 'negative self-evaluations and feelings of distress elicited by one's perceived failures or transgressions'. Causal guilt arises when someone feels guilty because they believe they are *causally* responsible for something that ought not to have happened. Adult children may ascribe their older parent's situation as being their fault, resulting in a feeling that they failed to do enough to care for their parent. They may feel causal guilt for moving a parent into a home, despite the inevitability of the move. I found that guilt can limit the capacity to provide care and to visit and this was evident amongst many of the adult child relatives. Fred (aged 56) noticed that his brother would find visits to the care home emotionally distressing and he would fall into this cycle of guilt which would in turn affect his ability to visit his parents.

> '[My brother] would go and drop in and see them, and he'd find it depressing, and he'd find it frustrating, and he'd come away feeling worse in himself, because they hadn't addressed anything that they could have chosen to. So, then that would put him off calling in next time. And then because he hadn't called in last time, and he didn't call in the next time, the next time he was passing he would feel even more guilty.'

Fred's brother noticed that things "hadn't been addressed" by the care home staff, which just added to his own sense of impotence, powerlessness, and guilt at the situation.

I found that there were two common responses to guilt: one was removing oneself from the situation, while the other was to become over-involved and to micro-manage a parent's care. Care home manager Tina recognised this and said, "sometimes the guilt of a relative can actually make them very anxious, but it can also make them become very critical":

> 'I think some people, because of their guilt, the only way that they feel they can show that they care is to come in and really analyse all of the care. Sometimes it's something within their psyche that if they say it's not been done quite right, it somehow helps them feel that they're doing something.'

Here the manager is highlighting how relatives felt a need to "show they care" by finding fault. It might be useful to consider again here Tronto's (1993) definition of 'caring about', which relates to recognising a need for care with the related moral value of *attentiveness*. In response to this, Lloyd (2012, p 39) cautions that although attentiveness is an important element in maintaining ethics of care, it is important to ensure that attentiveness does not become 'over-intrusive or a form of surveillance'. What we might recognise here is that guilt can result in a form of critical attentiveness when an adult child thinks that they are 'caring about' the needs of their parent.

The manager in this situation recognised that relatives needed additional reassurance and that maintaining a culture of openness and transparency in the home was part of this. She said, "It is about being very open with relatives who are complaining and saying 'Yeah, I'm really, really sorry. We're not getting this right, are we? How can we make it better? What would you like us to do to get it better?" She continued: "Which takes a certain amount of, dare I say, skill because it's very easy to become defensive if you feel like you're under attack." Garner (2004, p 221) writes 'the patient who does not get better may provoke feelings of aggression and sadism accompanied by anxiety, guilt, depression, and reparative wishes'. In the same way, an older parent in declining and terminal ill-health may provoke the same emotional responses. Impotent anxiety leads to attack as a defensive strategy, which includes positioning the staff or the care home as the 'enemy'. This can also result in over-involvement and meddling in a parent's care, with the attitude that staff are just not getting it right.

One care home manager said that they often spend more time reassuring the relatives rather than the resident on the first day of a move into her care home. She said, "It's the relatives, they're feeling great guilt, you know? 'Oh, but we've always looked after Mum, and I just can't do it no more', and 'I didn't want to put her in a place like this'." Volunteer Lydia also recognised the guilt involved in the move. She said, "I think there's a lot of guilt involved. The transition can be quite difficult for them." I asked, "Do you think that the guilt might prevent relatives from coming in?" She replied, "Yes, I do. Definitely. Yeah, I think that's probably a big thing, especially if their parent is anti-coming here, and they're saying, you know, 'Please don't put me in a home'. It must be dreadful. It must be absolutely dreadful, because obviously sometimes people can't cope." Care home manager Tina said, "Often there's a lot of guilt attached. People can feel dreadfully guilty about putting a relative in a home." Guilt can also be one of the main barriers to care home visiting and it is in the interests of the care home to ensure that adult children feel secure in their decisions to move their parent into care, and to support them in maintaining good relationships once they are in there.

When visits are forgotten

Adult children struggled with and questioned the usefulness of their visits to their parents in care, particularly when their parent had advanced dementia. Ruth (aged 54) described how her brother recently announced, "I've decided I'm not going to visit Dad any more on a Sunday because it's too difficult, and unpleasant, and he doesn't know who I am". This announcement caused significant conflict in her sibling group. Many relatives, however, found it challenging to visit their parents when conversations were repeated or there was little to talk about. Fred (aged 56) found it hard to visit his dad and he remembered asking "What have you been doing?" knowing that his dad had not been doing anything at all, so conversations turned to "Are you comfortable?" and "Have you got what you need?". Fred found these conversations difficult to maintain and cited this as a reason why he had rarely visited.

Relatives expressed frustration at the fact that their visits went unrecognised and there was often a mismatch between the visits that occurred and what was perceived to have happened by the older person. Lily (aged 57) described the balancing act that she had to find with visits to her mum. She said, "Sometimes she'll say, 'You haven't been for a while, have you?' and sometimes that's true, but sometimes I've been the day before. So, it is a difficult one – about how often you go." Sharon (aged 54) recalled how she spent from "1 o'clock till 6 o'clock there, and when she [her mother] rang me last night she didn't know I'd been". And Ruth (aged 54) told me, "You could go and spend half an hour with him, come out of the room for two minutes, go back, and he would not remember that you had just been with him". Volunteer Lydia told me how she supported an older lady who would cry "Oh, they don't come to see me because they're very busy". However, Lydia knew that the daughter visited regularly and took her mum out for day trips and walks, but that her mum would forget these visits and become resentful of her daughter. Maeve (aged 79), too, cried about her son not coming to see her. When interviewing her she said tearfully, "I am waiting for my son to come back, and he is supposed to come on Saturday but every time I look at the television it tells me it is Friday". I reminded her that it was indeed Friday today. She continued to cry, "He is never here. I do want him to come. I miss him so much."

Maeve spoke about her old home which she could see from her care home window. It had a "green gable and white bark trees" and her son lived there now. Maeve was a permanent resident in the home, but her old home, which was now up for sale, was within 100 yards of her window. Initially I thought it was nice that she could see her old home, but then realised that it might be quite hard to see it every day and might bring up painful memories for her. Although her son lived close by, they had fallen out and he never came to see her (something the care staff also told me). She cried, "He never visits me, and he only lives there. He only lives across the road." I did not meet Maeve's son so I could only wonder at the reasons why he might not visit very often. Perhaps he did and she had forgotten his visits? Perhaps he was too busy? Perhaps he felt safe in the knowledge that she was being looked after? Perhaps he felt guilty about her living there whilst he lived in her home? Perhaps he had his own physical or mental health struggles? Or perhaps he could not face witnessing his mother's declining health and what this might mean for her and for him. Care home manager Sheila noticed that if older parents were suffering from dementia, that their adult children would "feel that they're not recognised, and they find it hard, so they slowly come less and less". She observed, "It's the dementia that holds people back".

Geographical proximity and visiting

Geographical mobility in the UK, which is often a prerequisite for economic survival for many families, can lead to weak community bonds and can be an obstacle for family involvement in an older parent's care. Geographical proximity can be a predictor of involvement in older parent caregiving, and distance can sometimes be used as a reason not to be involved in care tasks or visits. Lily (aged 57) noticed that because she and her older sister were local to their mother's care home, that there was a (perhaps gendered) expectation and a 'judgement' in the sibling group that they should visit their mum every day and she was irritated that her siblings would monitor the signatures in the visitor's book to see when and how often she visited.

Older residents in the care homes were aware of the geographical distance between them and their children, and how this affected the level of contact that they had. Mildred (aged 86) said:

> 'I've got a daughter, as I said, but she lives in the North, and I haven't seen her for quite a while. I'm trying to think when it was, two years, easy. She came once when I'd just moved in. She says it's a long way, so. I know, it is a long way.'

I asked her how she felt about that. She replied:

> 'I couldn't describe how I feel. But it happens, doesn't it, when they move away? So, I just rely on my son. It's just one of those things. It happens in families, doesn't it? But I'm quite happy here, so I don't mind. It's just one of those unfortunate things.'

For some adult children, living a long way from the care home means that visiting is a real challenge, particularly when they have their own health needs or other responsibilities to attend to. Those visiting older people in care homes are sometimes of an advancing age themselves. Mildred's daughter, for example, was 67 years old and did not like to travel too much due to her own poor health. Another visitor that I met on one care home visit was in her 80s and visiting her centenarian mother. Deena, a care home manager, said: "I do have to remind staff as well that the relatives are actually quite old and can't always make it in here every day because they're old, and in ill-health and things like that, and sometimes that's why they're not in."

Many of the care home residents that I met did not have any family visitors at all. Some residents had no family left alive, some had never had children, and others had family who did not or could not visit. Some of the residents in the care home had suffered the loss of their own adult child. Penelope (aged 95) had lost her youngest daughter 18 months before I interviewed her. Reverend Dawson's (aged 86) daughter had died tragically in her early 40s. Maeve (aged 79) had three sons, but one had died aged 50 from a sudden heart attack. Betty (aged 86) did not have any children but had relied upon four nephews for her care prior to her move into the home, yet three of her four nephews had also now died.

There were many accounts of adult children being perceived as 'too busy' to visit. Peters et al (2006, p 544) found in their study of older parents' ambivalent perceptions of their relationships with their adult children, that 'parents preferred uncomplicated events and activities that allowed for meaningful conversation and time to just be together' and that 'it can be difficult to cultivate interactions experienced as quality time when children are busy'. Accounts from the older people I interviewed often told me that their adult children "have got their own lives to lead". Reverend Dawson said, "They claim to be so busy they can't do this, that, and the other." Elisabeth (aged 84) told me, "One of my sons lives in Scotland so I don't see him much, and the other one is in Kent. He's got his own business in Kent, so he's got his own life down there." I asked Maeve if anyone ever takes her out, and she replied "Yeah my children do, but it's not enough. They have got their own lives to lead." The volunteers I interviewed also noticed the busyness of the families and the residual guilt from this. Veronica, a volunteer, said, "People don't have time these days. They're all rushing around. It's almost an obligation for them to come in."

Some of the residents I interviewed were resentful about the lack of visits from their children. For instance, when interviewing Coral (aged 84) there was a sense of bitterness towards her daughter for putting her in a care home. This was our poignant exchange:

Bethany: Can you tell me, first of all, how you came to be here?
Coral: I wish I knew! My daughter gave up on me, I think is the only answer. I feel I've been put into a hotel for unwanted mothers.
Bethany: Were you living with your daughter before you came here?
Coral: No, I was living independently, but she was keeping an eye on me. And she suddenly decided she'd had enough, I suppose. I don't know.

She went on to say: "We together went through various places, and this seemed like the best of the worst." I did not get to speak to Coral's daughter to get her perspective on the situation, but Coral's thoughts about how she ended up in care could easily have resulted in making her daughter feel guilty about the decision and reluctant to visit.

Digital technology can help bridge some of the time and space divide between family members. The research data collection for this book was conducted prior to the COVID-19 pandemic, and the use of technology in care homes was not commonplace. Some residents received phone calls, but these were not always dialled through to the privacy of their own rooms. There were initiatives to provide older people with technology, such as iPads to help older people connect with their loved ones, but care home staff were often too busy (or technologically under-confident) to help set them up or assist with their use. The homes I visited usually had a single desktop in a central and public place in the care home such as in the lounge or conservatory, which was underused and often not even connected to the internet. Staff did not always know the passwords to access the computer and residents felt it was too much effort to use it.

However, the shielding of older, vulnerable care home residents, and the closure of care homes to external visitors during the COVID-19 pandemic, saw a necessary shift to the increasing use of digital communication with families. Adult children had to quickly adopt new ways of connecting with their parents. Lightfoot and Moone (2020) looked at 'the adaptive and emerging practices in formal supportive services for family caregivers, the changing types of support that family caregivers are providing to their older relatives, and the ways family caregivers are seeking informal caregiving support during the COVID-19 outbreak'. They found that telephone and/or video calls were now being used to supplement in-person visits and that this has become 'the main way many caregivers are staying connected with their relatives in community or long-term care settings' (Lightfoot and Moone, 2020, p 547). They found that this use of technology was a means to 'reduce the social isolation of older people who are not able to participate in their typical social activities' (Lightfoot and Moone, 2020, p 547).

Lightfoot and Moone (2020) found that when visiting was prohibited during the pandemic, care homes developed innovative ways of connecting families whilst also maintaining social distancing. This included 'window-greetings' where caregivers stand outside the window and either wave or talk on the phone with their older relatives. Some relatives drove their cars past the care facility and honked their horns, some sang to relatives who were stood on care home balconies, and they found that there was a return to letter writing and setting up pen pals with family members, friends, or grandchildren (Lightfoot and Moone, 2020, p 547).

If there are any 'positive outcomes' from the pandemic, it is hoped that one will be that it highlighted the need to engage more with communication technologies in care settings and that this use of technology will continue into the future. It is hoped that this will open up the possibilities for new ways of engaging care home residents, not only with their geographically dispersed or busy families, but with the wider community too. This can only be a positive step forward for re-linking connections between care home residents and their families.

Chapter summary

Despite the multiple challenges for older people living in their own home (and challenges for their informal caregivers) moving into long-term residential care is still not considered to be the '"home" of choice' (Gugliucci and Whittington, 2014). The transition to care raises a range of emotional, physical, financial, and social challenges. Furthermore, there are complex relational changes in the transition to care which positions older people under the agency of others.

Moving into a care home is unchartered territory for most people and there can be resistance from both the adult child and their parent as a result of negative stereotypes about care and the associated fears of frailty and dependency. The move can feel particularly daunting if the new home feels unfamiliar and uncertain. There are associated and anticipated losses with the transition to care, including feeling a loss of autonomy, independence, and moving away from your friends, family, and community. The older person may find themselves thrust (sometimes quite quickly or unexpectedly) into a new, unfamiliar environment and with people they do not know. For some, the move creates an unsettling sense of grief, loss, and resignation. There can be feelings of abandonment, especially if the older person does not fully understand why they have had to move or has resisted the transition to care. However, once settled, there can be feelings of acceptance or relief. The older person has to navigate making new friends, settling into a new living environment, and being on the receiving end of care tasks by unfamiliar people. As a result, the care space can become a struggle for autonomy, agency, and identity.

Living in a new care home takes a period of adjustment, and navigating relationships with others forms an important part of this process. In this chapter we explored three types of social connections – those with others living in the home, those with care staff, and those with visiting adult children. Stories from older people in care homes, as presented here, paint a picture of nurturing relationships in which residents look out for one another and a sense of 'being in this together'. However, they also point to fractious and frustrating relationships when communication is hindered by physical and mental deterioration, difficulties in navigating the spatial environment, and a reluctance to form meaningful relationships with others whose lives may be short-lived.

Visiting an older parent in care can be as equally rewarding and it can be difficult. For adult children, visits can trigger a range of complex emotions, from guilt, anxiety, and persecutory feelings towards the care home and the care team, to feelings of relief and security that a parent is finally being looked after and the burden of responsibility has now shifted. In cases when visits were quickly forgotten by the older parent, adult children felt their presence to be pointless and unappreciated. For some of these families, the visits became so unfulfilling that visits dwindled or stopped altogether. Guilt also held some relatives back from visiting, as they sought to protect themselves from such overwhelmingly difficult emotions. Adult children were better able to cope with these complicated feelings when they found meaningful and creative ways to engage with their parent and life in the home. Carmeli (2014, p 2) writes, 'when the caregiver benefits, so does the care recipient'. We found that it was still relatively common in care homes to view the adult child's role as a 'visitor', and this is a role often simply accepted by all parties. However, a greater incorporation of an adult child's caregiving role can really help them feel valued and useful in a time of great anxiety. Enabling relatives to be more active in care homes can make the visits feel more rewarding. How many relatives know that they are allowed to give their parent a bath? How many know whether they can take their parents out on trips? How many know that they can do an activity with their parent and include other residents in it too? Many relatives are at a loss at what to do on a visit, besides sitting and talking to their parent, who sometimes is unresponsive or does not recognise them. What is important is giving the adult child the confidence that their presence, however fleetingly remembered, is valued and important. An older parent with dementia might not remember the event but they may well remember the feelings that were evoked.

Geographical proximity was an often-cited reason for the sparsity of visits to relatives, but since COVID-19 there has been an uptake of communication technologies in homes which hopefully will help facilitate connections with distant relatives and the wider community.

Care homes can be a site of struggle when temporal and administrative regulations come into conflict with the individual needs of the residents. It is important for residents to be recognised as individuals with distinct needs, wishes, hopes, dreams, and interests. This is central to a 'person-centred care approach' and yet in the care home setting it exists in contrast to the homogenisation and routinisation that can creep in when busy carers are looking after people who need a lot of help. It is important, however, to recognise the socio-emotional complexities in the relationships with care staff. Contemporary debates on care home staffing highlight the problems of underpaid workers on exploitative contracts, working in high-pressure environments, and overwhelmed with responsibility. It is never helpful to criticise workers who are overworked, under-appreciated, and under-paid, as it fosters bad feelings, is demotivating, and raises emotional defences which inhibit good care.

The older people's narratives as presented here note frustrations but also an understanding of the pressures that care staff are under. Staff made valiant efforts to engage residents in enjoyable group activities, but it was the attention to detail and noticing 'the little things' that made the greatest difference to the everyday lives of the residents. Successful relationships with staff primarily arose when the older person was granted autonomy over the temporal rhythms that were important to the older person – such as being able to choose when to eat and when to go to bed. The recurring themes of what was important when settling into care included feeling safe and looked after, the immediacy of assistance, should it be needed, particularly in a medical emergency, socialising and companionship, the regularity of good quality meals, homeliness and cleanliness without the worry of having to do your own chores, meaningful activities, and the valued privacy of one's own room.

6

The loss of parents in later life

Existing literature on grief has frequently underplayed the psychological impact the loss of an older parent can have on the adult child. In this chapter we will turn our attention to the experience of loss which arises from witnessing the cognitive and physical decline of a parent's health, evoking fears for the parent's future and existential anxiety for the adult child. It will be argued that bereaved adult children experience a significant increase in psychological distress, a greater awareness of personal mortality, increased existential sensitivity, a reprioritisation of life goals, and a recalibration of relationships in the external world in the intra-psychic space. Furthermore, there is a significant experience of loss and a process of grieving which occurs before the physical death, and this is an experience which is commonly disenfranchised.

Timeliness and the disenfranchised death

Following the death of an older person, the bereaved are often 'comforted' with idioms or platitudes such as 'they had a good innings' or 'it was for the best', suggestive of a hierarchy of grief related to the 'timeliness' of the death. The death of an older parent is considered 'timely', and wider societal attitudes towards this type of loss are often disenfranchised (Marshall and Rosenthal, 1982; Osterweis et al, 1984; Moss and Moss, 1989; Scharlach and Fuller-Thomson, 1994; Taylor and Norris, 1995; Umberson, 1995; Smith, 1999). Timeliness refers to a death happening in the expected part of the life course, and the meaning and the consequences of the loss may differ by the timing of the death (Arbuckle and de Vries, 1995). For instance, the tragic death of a child may be considered to induce a greater sense of loss and distress compared to a natural death in the final stages of the life course (Calhoun et al, 2010). In comparison, the death of an older parent is frequently treated as a 'normative life event' (Scharlach and Fuller-Thomson, 1994) because the generational order dictates that the oldest generations die first. Taylor and Norris (1995, p 30) write that the 'death of a parent when you are middle-aged and your parent is elderly seems more part of the natural timing of events'. Consequently, the death of an older parent can be minimised or underplayed, making it difficult for the depth of grief to be fully acknowledged and worked through. Dying in a 'timely order' is used to deny the depth of emotional experience of the mourner.

Ken Doka's 1989 book, *Disenfranchised Grief*, highlighted that there were certain situations in life in which we can experience a sense of grief and loss, but these feelings are ignored or minimised. There is often a misunderstanding of the loss and a lack of understanding and appreciation of the depth of emotional suffering which people experience in these types of loss. Attig (2004, p 198) in his later text, 'Disenfranchised Grief Revisited', wrote that: 'Disenfranchising messages actively discount, dismiss, disapprove, discourage, invalidate, and delegitimate the experiences and efforts of grieving. And disenfranchising behaviours interfere with the exercise of the right to grieve by withholding permission, disallowing, constraining, hindering, and even prohibiting it.' He continues stating that: 'This misunderstanding of suffering actually compounds the loss and hurt that mourners endure. It induces and reinforces feelings of helplessness, powerlessness, shame, and guilt. And it withholds support from, breaks connections with, isolates, and abandons the bereaved in their sorrow' (Attig, 2004, p 205).

No one would doubt that the death of an older parent would elicit sympathy responses from those surrounding the adult child. And it is unlikely an adult child would be denied the opportunity to mourn the death – albeit there may be a societal expectation to come to terms with it sooner given its 'timeliness'. However, I found that the grieving process begins before the biological death occurs, and it is this grief which goes unrecognised, emotionally isolating the adult child. This grieving process, before death, arises as a result of 'anticipatory', 'progressive', and 'acknowledged' losses.

Types of loss

'Anticipatory loss' is a term coined by Pauline Boss in the 1970s, referring to a situation of loss which is unresolved, incomplete, or uncertain. In her later work (Boss, 1999) she identified two types of ambiguous loss. The first arises when it is unclear whether the person is still biologically alive, such in the case of a missing person. In this case the person is physically absent but psychologically present; their body is missing but they are held alive within the mind. In the second type of ambiguous loss, the person is physically present but psychologically absent, and this relates to witnessing a loved one with dementia for example. In this second typology, the physical body is present, but it is felt that the person within has been lost. In both forms of ambiguous loss, the relatives may grieve for their loved one whilst they are still living and over a long, gradual period of time (Dupuis, 2002, p 94). In the 1960s, Glaser and Strauss (1966) introduced the concept of the 'social death', which referred to how someone may appear to die socially and psychologically before their biological death. Králová (2015, p 237) writes that 'analysis of repeatedly occurring structural similarities in diverse studies of social death reveals three underlying notions: a loss of social identity, a loss of social connectedness and losses associated with disintegration of the body'.

Through the development of Boss's work, Dupuis (2002) recognised that there were other forms of 'non-death' loss which arise when relating to someone towards the end of their life. She writes about 'progressive loss', which refers to the witnessing of a gradual deterioration in health and/ or the disintegration of mental capacity of a loved one. Characterised by unpredictability and uncertainty about the future (Dupuis, 2002, p 101), the phase of progressive loss often begins in the mid-phase of the institution-based caregiving career and involves living through and dealing with the gradual loss of loved ones (Dupuis, 2002, p 102). Progressive loss can be correlated with ambiguous loss and refers to a 'loss situation that remains incomplete, confusing, or uncertain for family members' (Dupuis, 2002, p 94). It is this uncertainty and incompleteness which poses the challenge for the adult child. They may be experiencing deep grief but are unable to mourn openly, constituting a form of disenfranchised grief.

Ambiguous loss was evident in adult children's stories of their parents' declining health. Lily (aged 57) said about her mum:

'I'm not saying I want her to die now, but when she does die, of course it's going to be difficult. It's almost as if you have sort of been through a lot of that because that person, that relationship, that mother, is sort of gone really, and what's left is almost like a caricature, almost like a, not a skeleton, but sort of a, just an outline of that person that says and does some of the things that she used to say.'

Coleen (aged 45) described her father's health in a similar way, saying:

'He's got all these tablets basically keeping him alive, but the dementia is slowly, and the light's gone. And, and this is a controversial thing, and I will say it, but I'm just wondering, where do you get to the stage where you keep propping someone up with these tablets, when there's nothing left – they're almost an empty shell.'

Both accounts reveal confusion about the incompleteness of the loss of their parent. The language they use is telling: "skeleton", "empty shell", "an outline" are striking metaphors for someone considered dead whilst still physically alive.

Dupuis (2002) writes that 'acknowledged loss' is the recognition that a loved one no longer exists in the same way, and never will again. She found that the two most commonly use coping strategies for acknowledged loss were 'acceptance and avoidance' (Dupuis, 2002, p 93). In the avoidance strategy, family members might psychologically protect themselves from the loss by avoiding their loved one, reducing or ceasing visits to them in care, not inviting them to join in family events, not acknowledging their parent's role identity, and even talking about their parent as if they are already dead. There is a psychological retreat from the relationship. This was evident in Ruth's (aged 54) description of the relationship with her father. "He's still here. I'm still glad he's here, but he's not who he was. He was my rock." Towards the end of the interview, I asked how her father's move into care had affected her, and she replied: 'It was a really sad time, and that's the bit about losing both parents." She quickly corrected herself, "but clearly I have not lost my dad". This mis-saying "losing both parents" was an interesting slip of the tongue, revealing an unconscious belief that her father has already been lost. For Lily, witnessing her mother's weakening physical and mental health meant that she was considered less and less 'alive' – to the point where Lily had to reassure herself that her mum was still here. She said, "It's weird that I'm trying to reassure myself, 'No, she hasn't died'."

In the coping strategy of acceptance, relatives may have reached a pivotal moment in the ambiguous loss grieving process. At this point there is a psychological maturation and a 'coming to terms' with the loss. There is peace and acceptance of the changes in their loved one, and an acknowledgement that things will not ever return back to how they once were.

However, adult child may find themselves oscillating between different psychological positions of acceptance and avoidance. Adult children presented contradictory wishes for their older and frail parents to die, but also a deep wish for them to stay alive too. Coleen (aged 45) exemplified this, confessing:

'I know this is a really brutal thing to say, and these are the conversations I have with other people, where they say, "Well, they wouldn't let a dog live like that", but we have this thing where we have this fear of dying. We have this, the NHS has to keep people alive under whatever the circumstances. We have the fear of euthanasia. I almost think – and I don't want him to pass away, God Almighty, I really don't! I actually like the idea that he's still alive, because I often feel like I'm almost too young to have lost both my parents.'

If the burden of care for an older parent has been prolonged or particularly difficult then there can be relief at the parent's death due to the end of suffering for the parent but also due to the end of care duties. Sprang and McNeil (1995, p 22) wrote that 'society tends to be impatient with prolonged bereavement … the old are expected to die'. Perhaps then there is a truth in the feelings of impatience, which in turn make the adult child feel guilty and ashamed for entertaining those thoughts. This was most evident in Jeff's story. Jeff (aged 48) had a heavy care responsibility for his mother, and he felt he needed his mother to die in order for him to start leading a life of his own. Jeff's father had died of cancer when he was 5 years old, and Jeff's mother had struggled with severe mental health problems ever since. Now in her 80s, Jeff's mother was in very poor physical and mental health, and Jeff and his sister had cared for her for their entire lives. Neither had lived away from their mother and neither had formed a serious romantic relationship with anyone, had never had children, and Jeff had never been able to achieve his main life ambitions. He talked about his ambivalent feelings concerning his mother's death. In many ways he wanted her to die, but then found himself shifting to a fear of her dying. He said:

> 'I suppose I want her to die really. I mean I will be sad. I will be sad in some ways, and I think I've purposely distanced myself from the emotional bond sometimes. I think people are very flexible. I could easily find myself getting back into more of a sort of son/mother relationship and being terrified of her dying.'

Jeff could not separate himself from his child-like role. Despite having lived with and been the carer for his mother all his life, his mother was still his mother, and he was still her son. His roles were confused; his caring parenting role, his vulnerable child role, and his grown-up independent adult role were all conflicted with one another. He had a deep desire to grow up and be independent, but he also had a fear of separation. Coleen, Lily, and Jeff all narrated this parallel emotional experience of feeling that a parent had lived 'too long', yet retained a deep longing for them to stay alive. There is also a child-like distress in their stories. Jeff's 'terror' of losing his son/mother relationship and Coleen's cry of "I'm almost too young to have lost both my parents" perhaps are reflective of their rejection of an impending new identity as a midlife orphan and the implications this has for their own ageing process and mortality awareness.

When faced with the terminal decline of an older parent, particularly towards the very end of life, the adult child may not know which of their visits is their last. They recognise that every significant health change could signify the end. Being faced with an irreconcilable and imminent loss is an emotionally exhausting experience. It leaves the family and the older person to deal with deep existential questions about the life that has been led and the death that is to come. There is an unpredictability about this liminal space between life and death. Lily said, "They call it 'the long goodbye', and I feel like I did a lot of that 'good-byeing' when she first started going downhill, and when she went into the home, and then it seemed like we've lost so much of her" and she continued, "you just don't know when it's going to happen". Dupuis (2002, p 109) also writes about this long and painful grieving process as the 'long good-bye' and 'the never-ending funeral'. And with progressive loss, changes in a parent may be evident with every visit. They may be cognitively aware in one visit but absent in the next. This not knowing what will happen next and what the appropriate emotional response should be causes great stress upon the adult child relative.

Ambiguous and progressive loss is particularly confusing, painful, and overwhelming, because the loss is repeated over and over again. With these multiple, sequential, and seemingly insignificant smaller losses which happen with the progressive loss of a parent, the accompanying grief is disenfranchised and does not elicit the same level of loss empathy from social support networks. Losses, before the final death, cannot be easily and openly mourned, and adult children are expected to carry on with life until the death happens (Smith, 1999, p 43). Adult children are expected to continue with work, family roles, and the tasks of everyday life without the opportunity to take time for a period of grief and reflection. The impact of these multiple losses can further lead to bereavement overload and weaken emotional resilience (Moss and Moss, 1996, p 27).

However, for some adult children when a parent does die physically, much of the grieving process will have already been worked through due to the processing of these multiple preceding losses. Hazel described her mother's death in a care home, following a period of dementia. She said: "To be frank and honest, she'd had a long life, and when she died, of course I was upset, but I didn't mind. ... But it is, there's a loss, so you mind that. But the loss was already there. It's just an extra loss." Joe (aged 49), too, recalls how he was not particularly emotional at his mother's funeral and that the only time he became upset was when he realised that he had lost his mum a long time before her actual death. He remembered: "I said after she died 'it's the only time I nearly got a bit tearful' and I said 'you know that's not my mum, because I don't think she had been my mum for a while'."

Just as Dupuis (2002) recognised that acknowledged loss included experiences of 'acceptance and avoidance', Freud's early work (1917) suggested that the threat of an impending death can generate a psychological detachment from the relationship in order to protect from the final loss and to deal more effectively with the rising anticipatory grief. Freud (1917) called this a process of 'decathexis', whereby the libidinal energy is removed from the loved object. According to Freud, this mourning process involves 'severing' each attachment one has to the loved object. Freud wrote that 'mourning occurs under the influence of reality-testing; for the latter demands categorically from the bereaved person that he should separate himself from the object, since it no longer exists' (1917, p 172). Freud wrote that in the process of mourning 'each single one of the memories and expectations in which the libido is bound to the object is brought up and hypercathected, and detachment of the libido is accomplished in respect of it … when the work of mourning is completed the ego becomes free and uninhibited again' (1917, p 245). Freud's (1917) early work, followed later by Bowlby (1961) and then Parkes (1972, 1975), all claimed that the goal of the mourning process is to lead to a detachment from the lost loved object. We might suggest that this is one explanation for some adult children refusing to visit their parents in care, and the seemingly callous need for detachment from their parents. This process of detachment from the loved parent protects the adult child from imminent pain and ultimate loss.

Freud later reconsidered this early theory on complete detachment, instead suggesting (in his text 'The Ego and the Id', 1923) that there follows a process in which libidinal energy is displaced and reattached to a new loved object in the form of a substitute, for example the adult child putting all their energy into another relationship (a romantic relationship, work, or children), or into a new relationship with the lost parent. Klass et al's (1996) *Continuing Bonds: New Understandings of Grief* challenged these earlier linear models of grief which suggested that acceptance and detachment from the lost loved object were the goals. Instead, they recognised the importance, and normalcy, of promoting a continued bond with the deceased. And it is through these continuing bonds that the bereaved can gain comfort, resilience, and adjustment. Foote et al (1996, p 150) recognised that it is 'possible and helpful to have a continuing relationship with the person who died'. They write that 'the challenge is to discover new and constantly changing ways of taking the dead person along on the rest of one's journey through life' (1996, p 150). Angell et al (1998, p 618) write that contemplating, fantasising, and dreaming of a lost parent is a spiritual process which locates our parents in 'a time and place and transporting our recreated experiences to the here-and-now'. This may take the form of an internal dialogue with the idealised parental figure in their inner world. In that psychic space, roles can be reversed, and the parent–child relationship cognitively restored. Shmotkin (1999, pp 478–9) recognised the continuing bonds with dead parents and that adult children continued to be 'occupied and influenced by the parents' imaginary presence and emotional impact' and that in the process of bereavement there was a 'restructured relationship and revitalized engagement with the inner representation of the lost person'. Shmotkin (1999, p 480) further suggests that 'these powerful bonds go beyond normative mourning, extend the past connection into the present separation, and continue to resonate family constellation and roles'. Continuing dialogue with a dead parent serves the important function of reconfiguring roles and relationships, returning thoughts to the familiar when life feels disrupted, and anchoring memories in the mind. In her study on the death of parents, Umberson (2003) also recognised the importance of a belief in the afterlife in comforting the bereaved and allowing them to understand that the deceased parents is not permanently lost to them. She writes, 'The parent plays such a powerful role in shaping the child's sense of self that the parent can be said to reside within the child throughout life' (2003, p 82).

It is important to note that this reconnection with a lost loved one does not have to be as the result of a religious belief, or even necessarily a spiritual belief. It may be achieved through a variety of symbolic forms, firstly such as generative achievements and the creation of a legacy, or through creative endeavours such as art, writing, or telling stories that have been passed on. It might be through rituals such as tree planting or funding a prize in their name.

Reminiscence and preoccupation are powerful aspects of the grieving process. Remembering is the ability to bring memories into the present conscious awareness and helps connect the living with those who have died. It helps the mourner to recognise the legacy that their loved one has left behind and this helps forge that connection beyond their physical death. Attig (2004, p 213) writes that:

> The legacies of memory itself include moments, episodes, periods, and stories of their lives filled with enduring meanings not cancelled by death, meanings that themselves 'give life to life.' Remembering connects mourners with some of the best of life. It is itself an expression of their enduring love for those they mourn.

The preoccupation phase is an opportunity to reconnect with the lost object through intense mental absorption into thoughts about a lost parent. Petersen and Rafuls (1998, p 508) write about a preoccupation period in the grieving process in which they found that the bereaved adult child dealt with thoughts of their parent's death 'quietly internally, and without sharing, with the deepest meaning and purposes of life'. They found that their participants 'were somewhat unaware of how preoccupied they had been until someone else brought it to their attention' (1998, p 508). This was most evident in Hazel's (aged 68) account of how she had lost interest in everyday pleasures and a loss of concentration following her mother's death. She told me:

> 'I think there's a number of things about grief that I hadn't ever considered, because when my dad died, I had to look after my mum, and this time I've only got to look after myself. My sleep pattern has changed. I'm not interested in food. I mean, I'll sit and eat a meal, but I couldn't give a toss. I am used to reading a book every three or four days, it's taking me four weeks to read a book now. I'm not, I can't concentrate on what I'm reading, even if it's fascinating, right? I have to read it again. It's like my head's too full. I'm forgetting words.'

Hazel's account is particularly interesting here in that she describes a greater depth of grief following her second parent's (her mother's) death. Marshall (2004, p 361) described the death of parents in later life as a 'two-phased transition', with two distinct periods of mourning – one following the first parent and one following the second.

The order of parental death and the midlife orphan

Following the death of the first parent, adult children can experience a heightened awareness of their own mortality and the mortality of their remaining parent. There is a grief for the lost parent, and a changed relationship, sympathy, concern, and even grief on behalf of the remaining parent. Sometimes the adult child's grief is suppressed by the grief of the remaining parent, leading to changes in that relationship, perhaps an increase in responsibility, a change in roles, or additional concern for the welfare of the remaining parent. Once one parent dies and the other remains, this can create a double bind of grief. Marshall (2004, p 359) describes this as where 'an individual grieves both with, for, and alongside another person'. Furthermore, the adult child may modify their grieving process so that they appear strong or resilient in front of their remaining parent.

Marshall (2004, p 362) noticed that it was only following the death of a second parent that adult children felt permitted to 'own' their grief. Diane (aged 55) recognised that she had not had the opportunity to process the loss of her dad alongside her mum's intense grief. She said:

> 'I mean she's never been to my dad's grave since he passed away. I think to this day she can't accept it, even though it's nine years on, ten actually. I find it very difficult sometimes to talk about my dad. I have to be careful you know what I say sometimes. I don't want to upset her, and she won't have flowers in the house, not since the funeral.'

Joe (aged 49) described that once his dad had died his mother became "a sub person" with "no role in life" – "She had no function at all." In an ageing spousal relationship, the husband and wife often support each other through age-related challenges, and there is usually a division of labour with household tasks. However, when one parent dies the care requirements of the remaining parent may increase, as that form of support is no longer available at home. Fred (aged 56) noticed a distinct change in his parents' relationship as they got older, and how their needs increased, ultimately becoming more dependent upon one another.

> 'I do remember distinctly seeing Mum and Dad going from one phase of life where, yeah, they were in their 70s, to a new phase of life where

they both sort of realised they needed each other. And it was, it wasn't that they needed each other in a very loving way, but they realised they needed each other. So, there was a definite shift into a phase of their lives when they realised, subconsciously, I mean, they didn't verbalise it, but they needed each other.'

The death of the first parent may serve as a stark reminder about the care level requirements which may have gone under-recognised until this point. Hazel recalled:

'My dad died when she [mum] was almost 80 and since then I've had all the responsibility. I mean she'd never paid a bill and she'd never written a cheque. She hadn't had the responsibility of dealing with the state, or the gas company. She'd open these things, and she'd say, "What's this?" I said, "That's called the council tax". "Oh, will you pay it?" I'd reply "Of course". She didn't know how to do a lot of things, not because she was 80, but because my dad had always done them.'

This highlighted for Hazel (aged 68) the new, and advanced levels of care needs her mum required now that her dad had gone. In other examples, the death of the first parent revealed new characteristics, personality traits, and strengths that had previously been overshadowed. For example, Lisa (aged 45) found that following her father's death she was surprised by her mother's strength. "I think she's probably got a personality we didn't realise she had, she's a lot stronger than she thought she was and as I said, she was very much in my dad's shadow."

Marshall (2004, p 364) writes that the 'the second stage to the parent loss life transition involves reflection on a status as "parentless"' and that 'bereaved adult children may feel a sense of being an orphan'. Anna (aged 46) said that with the death of our parents, "we lose our sense of being a child". And a 56-year-old relative of my own once cried to me, "I am now an orphan", after having lost both of her parents within six months of each other.

In 1988 Bowlby introduced the idea that a secure and responsive attachment in a parental relationship provides the child with a 'secure base' as they develop. This secure base gives the child the space to venture into their surroundings with confidence. The child begins to learn what is dangerous in their external environment and they become more confident in their own abilities to do things for themselves, developing self-sufficiency and a sense of individual identity. Bowlby (1988, p 62) writes 'All of us, from the cradle to the grave, are happiest when life is organised as a series of excursions, long or short, from the secure base provided by our attachment figures'. Yet, when our parents (our once secure base) reach the end of life or die they no longer provide that sense of security for that child-like part of ourselves.

McDaniel and Clark (2009, p 45) state, 'when the last parent dies, there is no "home" for the child to return to. The parents are dead. Relationships, however, never die.' Pritchard writes that 'the loss of a parent evokes all the old fears and threats of the lost child' (1995, p 153). Archer argued that to lose a parent in adulthood is 'difficult to cope with because they make the individual's personal world an unsafe and unpredictable place' (1999, p 213). Just as a child first ventures from the security of its primary caregiver, so too must the adult child renegotiate the world around them alone following both their parents' deaths. Although aspects of this separation process from parents are reminiscent of earlier infantile experiences, it is now experienced in a qualitatively different way. Jaques (1965, p 505) suggested that one of the differences between earlier infantile experiences of loss and of those experienced in midlife is that midlife 'calls for a re-working through of the infantile depression, but with mature insight into death and destructive impulse to be taken into account'. Now in adulthood the child faces the ultimate and final loss of their parents and there is no option for the adult child to revert back to the child role.

Shmotkin (1999, p 474), however, cautions against comparisons between orphanhood at a young age and normative orphanhood in adult life, in that adult orphanhood has more possibility for growth and individuation. McDaniel and Clark (2009, p 45) claim that the death of the second parent raises a unique set of feelings and experiences. It is a 'maturing experience' as Silverman (1987) puts it, and is about relearning the world. Attig (1996, pp 13–14) writes that it is a period of the life course in which 'we find and make ways of living with our emotions and struggle to re-establish self-confidence, self-esteem, and identity in a biography colored by loss'. Petersen and Rafuls (1998, p 512) quoted a woman who had lost both parents as saying, 'something in me grew up'. Having a connection with a supportive and protective parent gives the adult child a sense of belonging and a place to return to in times of need. Even if that relationship is more complicated, that loss can still be felt deeply as the hope for an improved or idealised connection with a parent is also lost.

New roles and responsibilities

When a parent dies physically or psychologically, family roles are reassigned and personal identities are reconfigured. If the parent was in a position of leadership within the family, then leadership responsibilities may be passed on through continuing family traditions or keeping continuity of a parent's legacy. McDaniel and Clark (2009, p 45) write that 'maintaining or ending family traditions is now one of many responsibilities and choices required of the surviving adult children'. Petersen and Rafuls (1998, p 500) call this 'accepting the scepter', writing that: 'The emergent theme was of passing the sceptre of roles and responsibilities previously held by the deceased parent to the next generation of the grieving adult child. Respondents assumed the responsibility of "making things right for the future generations of the family'" (Petersen and Rafuls, 1998, p 501).

An interesting observation from my research was the internal change in some bereaved adult children who have not only adopted their deceased parent's roles and responsibilities, but also have begun emulating their personal characteristics. Shmotkin (1999, p 479) termed this a form of 'idealization', writing, 'idealization reflects a selective adoption of positive attributes in the deceased figure, so that the internal representation of the deceased continues to sustain meaningfulness and reassurance for the bereaved person.' Adult children described moments in which they found themselves imitating their lost parent or fearing that they were turning into them. Hazel described how she "can't remember things" following the death of her mother through dementia, and how "this has got worse" since she had died. Another adult child found that in times of anxiety she would clap her hands together, almost as a tic, which was the same motion her mother had developed as her dementia had advanced. We might suggest that this behaviour arises due to the psychologically confronting nature of the parental death and that 'witnessing a parent's death means witnessing the death of a part of oneself' (Umberson, 2003, p 17), and that developing a parent's character serves to keep not only the parent psychologically alive, but also keeps a part of oneself alive too.

Difficult parental relationships

Much of the discussion so far has focused on relatively congenial relationships with older parents. However, it is important to acknowledge those parent–child relationships which are complicated, ambivalent, distant, or dysfunctional. Most family relationships have some level of dissonance, and this can be complicated if care decisions have to be made for, and with, older parents with whom the relationship is less than harmonious. The death of a parent when there is a difficult relationship can lead to an experience of traumatic grief. Petersen and Rafuls (1998, p 508) write that 'the grieving process was more disruptive in those families with dysfunction and conflict prior to the death'. They suggest that the more dysfunctional the relationship was prior to the death, the more complicated and long lasting the grief process was after it. One of the key complicating factors in this grieving process is the loss of hope that one day the parent may change and become the parent that you had longed and hoped for (Umberson, 2003, p 65); this is the loss of possibility. Another factor is that when someone dies there tends to be an idealisation of their character with their flaws being ignored. The mourner has to come to terms with both the positive and negative aspects of the deceased's character in the company of others who may be celebrating their life. A further complicating factor is a sense of relief and then the guilt that can follow that. Petersen and Rafuls (1998, p 513) write that 'freedom from the dysfunctional "hold" parents had on their adult children was an unforeseen gift in the aftermath of the death' and that 'in those families where dysfunction was a serious issue, liberation from those patterns on the death of the parent provided motivation, hope for change, and empowerment to implement the change' (Petersen and Rafuls, 1998, p 518). Similarly, Taylor and Norris (1995, p 31) claimed that some people experienced the bereavement of a dysfunctional parent as 'a welcome severing of destructive family ties that provides an opportunity for growth unhampered by parental expectations'. Relief following the death of a parent is also a complicated grief response, often resulting in feelings of guilt and shame. Given that there is often an intense caregiving burden and emotional strain upon the adult child preceding the death of an older parent, it is not surprising that some adult children felt a sense of relief and liberation from that experience. Bernard and Guarnaccia (2003, p 810) describe a 'relief model of bereavement' which proposes that caregivers frequently experience caregiver strain. Once caregiving obligations end with the death of the care recipient, there can be an experience of post-death caregiver relief, and this provides the opportunity to re-establish previously neglected roles in employment, family, and in leisure time.

As described earlier, Jeff lost his father to cancer when he was a 5-year-old. In terms of psychosexual development, this could be significant in that it appeared as if Jeff had triumphed in his primitive oedipal phantasy (Freud, 1900). As a young child Jeff may have felt in some way responsible for his father's death and guilt that he now had his mother all to himself – and indeed as an adult he lived his life *as if* he was married to his mother. His mother's behaviour seemed to enforce this by not allowing him to leave or have romantic relationships or friendships. Their relationship seemed exclusive and insular, based on guilt, love, and fear. Jeff spoke of being "trapped" and often dreamt of a life without his mother. He considered plans for the future but did not think they could be realised until his mother had died:

'I am at home looking after my mother. I still have ideas of moving in with people, but it doesn't seem practical at the moment…The fact that my mum's health has stabilised might mean that she lives for another ten years or more when in fact last year I thought that she couldn't last the year. So that affects things practically.'

Jeff spoke candidly about the phantasy of his mother dying and the brief excitement he felt when he thought she would die:

'For my mother's health, one of the GPs diagnosed that my mother had bowel cancer from the blood tests, and this was about a year back and I suddenly thought I had a thrill go through me, that this is an escape, an escape for me from all this being tied down – not being able to go on holidays and things like that. But it's an escape for Mum from all the pain and all the other things that she has to go through. But of course, the GP got it wrong, so it was nothing of the kind [laughs] I suppose that's a good test reaction to Mum.'

It is interesting that Jeff is unapologetic about this reaction. I suggest that the passage into adulthood was something which both intrigued Jeff and was something to fantasise about but at the same time it also frightened him, and he retreated into the security of being close to his mum through her care. He told me, "I'm quite trapped in a way. There's lots of things I can't do. Then again, that makes life less stressful in certain ways," indicating that his limited life opportunities also protected him from other pressures.

Jeff was torn between a loyalty towards his mother and a realisation that his own life was passing him by. He was also split by the security he felt with her and his need for autonomy and independence. He fluctuated between the different emotions, suggestive of being in what Klein (1946) termed the paranoid schizoid position. Roth states that, 'as adults we can retreat to a paranoid-schizoid state of mind when we are threatened by too much anxiety, or by illness, or by traumatic events' (2005, p 52). Psychological splitting is a primary feature of this paranoid schizoid position, and Jeff certainly had split feelings about his situation and relationship with his mother. Throughout the interview he fluctuated between the Kleinian 'good breast' of the security providing mother, and the 'bad breast' of the mother who controls his life and holds him back. It is perhaps the guilt he felt about the psychological attack on the bad elements which ultimately kept him in a reparative state of trying to make his mother better, and his prolonged care role. Also, by focusing his energies on her dependence on him, he did not have to confront his own dependence on her. This kind of behaviour by Jeff could be seen as a psychological defence. By wishing his mother dead he did not have to face the loss in its full and devastating entirety, instead he devalued the loved object (his mother), helping to make the final loss psychologically easier to cope with.

Chapter summary

The death of a parent represents a critical attachment loss, with the relationship with a parent being our most enduring relationship (Douglas, 1990, in Sprang and McNeil, 1995, p 21). Following such a loss the adult child's identity is irrevocably changed through a process of adaptation to, and emotional integration of, the loss of the symbolic figure who has been there – in a functional relationship – since infancy.

On a societal level the death of an older parent is considered normative and timely, resulting in a disenfranchisement and minimisation of the emotional pain that accompanies such a loss. Yet the death of a parent can result in a painful loss, almost inconceivable in its magnitude, and one which taps into a deep, primitive level of existential anxiety.

The loss of a parent can reawaken old threats, anxieties, and defences which were first experienced in the early infantile stages. Feelings of abandonment and threats to attachment, juxtaposed by the need for independence and autonomy, are the original dilemmas of infancy but are replayed in midlife with a new understanding of death. This stage of the life course is about recognising the revised position in the generational hierarchy, that independence from parents is a necessary part of being grown up. The threatened and impending loss of parents, however, is often overwhelming and the state of anticipatory mourning can create a range of different psychological reactions, including psychic attacks to sever the psychological ties with a loved one in order to deal more effectively with the anticipatory sense of grief, and this has significant consequences for how older parents are then cared for at the end of life.

Prolonged illness and a prolonged dying process can result in 'psychosocial death' (Doka and Aber, 1989, p 189; Dupuis, 2002, p 94), involving a loss of self, connection, and identity. And although this may be true for some, it is important to recognise that social relations can still remain alive and present for others; families can still remain active in the lives of older people with advanced dementia or other progressive illnesses. It is also important for care facilities and staff to encourage person-centred narratives, to promote inclusionary practices even with those at the very end of life, and to involve families in maintaining social relationships and helping to keep their parent 'socially alive'.

Final reflections

Whilst much research has been undertaken to explore the experiences of older people and how to improve their quality of life, far less attention has been paid to the psychosocial experiences of their adult children who are often tasked with difficult decisions about care provision and arranging a parent's affairs. Emerging from this research is a complexity of emotional responses to the caregiving experience for adult children. Adult children can feel a sense of responsibility and duty towards the care of parents, along with compassion, commitment, and increased emotional bonds. However, there can also be conflicting, and painful, emotional responses such as frustration, resentment, guilt, and loss which also need to be acknowledged.

The psychosocial research methodology underpinning this research has been used to uncover some of the more difficult or taboo discussions about the relationship with older parents. I once gave a conference presentation in which I introduced Jeff's story about his difficult relationship with his mother. Some audience members were aghast at Jeff's admission that he had sometimes wished for his mother's death in order to live a more fulfilled life. This was not something to be talked about. Yet he was not the first, nor the last to admit such difficult emotions when faced with very challenging care relationships. Although it was a difficult thing for Jeff to admit, it also highlighted the psychologically conflicting care role that he and many other adult children face. This is not to deny the love and care in those relationships, but instead it highlights the emotional struggles, or ambivalence, that adult children can feel in their caregiving experiences.

This book introduced the concept of the 'generational shift', which sees the upward movement of the generations, which for the midlife adult child means the ageing and loss of the generations above, as well as changes in the generations below. There are competing demands from multiple directions – children, career, own psychical and mental health, marriage, managing a home and the affairs of a parent's home, as well as loss, grief, and anxiety about a parent's ageing, choosing a care home, coping with guilt, and arbitrating other family and sibling relationships; all gather pace at this point in the life course. But it is this generational shift that, I argue, can raise existential anxiety and increase personal mortality awareness. It signifies the shifting of time and makes the midlife adult child more aware of their life stage. One of the big changes that highlights this shift is the move towards caring for an ageing parent. Providing care can change the child–parent relationship. An adult child may feel that they have become their parent's parent, particularly when there are intimate care tasks to be performed. Roles have reversed and whereas once they were a son or daughter to their parent, they now find themselves a carer, and this shift in role and identity can be deeply unsettling.

Adult children and their parents can both feel a sense of frustration and anxiety when there is a disparity between what care a parent needs and what they are willing to accept. In particular, if dementia is one of the reasons for the increase in care needs, the older parent may not recognise their need for support and can reject their adult child's offers of help. Adult children, when first faced with a parent whose health has rapidly deteriorated, can be conflicted about their role and how to relate to their parent. Adult children may be driven to care through a sense of duty and reciprocity – "mum did this for me, so I should do it for her", but equally there can be a rejection of this if the earlier parental role was not as nurturing as it could have been. This book illustrated how care tasks are distributed within the family systems, particularly amongst siblings. This coordination amongst siblings can be well organised and cooperative, with siblings recognising their skills and strengths, and admitting their weaknesses. In other sibling dynamics, this distribution of care tasks can be difficult, fraught with tensions which are often repetitions of older, infantile-based conflicts.

We considered the transitions and trajectories into care. Physical and mental health decline (acute and chronic conditions), loneliness, struggling to cope at home, and the inability of adult children to continue to provide care in the home were all reasons why an older parent might need to make a decision about increasing their level of support at home and eventually a move into care.

We saw that role of informal caregiving by adult children was often overlooked and the anticipatory grief that they felt when caring for an older parent was disenfranchised. Adult children often have competing demands of paid work, whilst caring for their own children (and/or grandchildren) and also caring for their older parents. This scenario is becoming more commonly referred to as the problems of the 'sandwich generation'.

When care responsibilities become too much to bear, decisions need to be made for additional long-term support. Yet, talking to a parent about a transition into a care home is another challenge. We saw that some parents were insulted by the suggestion, or resistant to the move, particularly if they themselves did not recognise that they were not coping as well as they used to. Resistance also arises in response to negative perceptions about what care homes are like. There is ongoing work that needs to be done to improve the perceptions of care homes. The My Home Life England initiative is one example of promoting appreciative enquiry into good care home practices and connecting up care homes with local communities. This opens care homes up to showing what life can be like in care, and modelling what good things are possible.

Moving a parent into a care facility is a courageous decision and involves enormous upheaval for both parent and child. For the adult child, one of the key tasks is managing the house and possessions that have been left behind. House clearance is a physically demanding task and is emotionally unsettling. Often older parents' homes contain sentimental possessions and associated memories, which all have to be sorted through and emotionally processed; each item uncovered representing a little loss. Whilst sorting the items, decisions have to be made about which are to be distributed amongst family, which are to be stored, which are to be sold or donated, and which are to be taken to the care home. We heard from some of the voices of older people and their experience of moving into a care home. Choice over what possessions they can take with them to the home, and what clothing they wear once they are there, are often decisions made for them. These physical objects play an important role in creating and maintaining a sense of identity, and help the older person settle into their new environment. Autonomy over space and time within the care home setting is also important for the older person – what time they go to bed, where they sit in the lounge or for dinner, how they structure their day, what they eat, who visits, and what activities are available to them are all important elements of care home life. Relationship building is also key to settling into a home. Making friends with other residents is important but can also be challenging when communication is hindered by mobility, sensory disabilities, or cognition changes. Feeling comfortable with care staff is important too, and these relationships can be compassionate, nurturing, and flourishing. However, if there is high staff turnover, or a culture of underappreciating, understaffing, and underpaying staff, levels of staff morale may be low, they may feel under pressure, and the connection to residents may suffer as a result.

Activity provision is an important part of care home life, but care needs to be taken in ensuring the appropriateness of the entertainment and tasks. It is also important to recognise why the activity is being facilitated: Is it because that is what the older residents want? Or is it because that is what the care home staff think older people want? The expectation to be 'doing something', I argue, is generationally loaded. We heard some of the voices of older people who "did not want to *do* anything!" Yet, if the activities are targeted to the needs, wants, and wishes of the older person, then they can be fun, joyful, and increase well-being. It was the 'little things' that made the most difference; attending to the small and frustrating things, like ensuring that they have the right cutlery, adjusting the flowers, or making sure they have their cup of tea made 'just right', can make all the difference to the day in the life of an older person living in care. These little things need to first be noticed, though, and in a culture of busyness in care homes, sometimes these things can be missed.

We have explored the experiences of visiting a parent in care from both the older parent and the adult child's perspectives. Adult children sometimes struggled to visit their parent for a number of reasons: competing family demands, having to work, geographical distance, their own advancing age and health needs, and more recently COVID-19 restrictions. Psychologically, visiting a parent can also be difficult. Visits may feel unfulfilling or pointless, especially if the parent doesn't remember it, or when a parent chastises an adult child for not visiting (when the child actually has visited but it has been forgotten). This can make the adult child not want to visit, increasing a sense of guilt and shame. However, if visits feel rewarding, welcoming, and supported by care staff then child–parent relationships can thrive and become even closer once the care burden has been lessened at home.

The final chapter of this book acknowledged the loss of parents in later life. It showed that the life course is experienced as a series of losses, but it is loss and its associated mourning that are required for deep psychological growth. Here we explore some of the models of grief from the literature and take a closer look at Dupuis' (2002) and Boss' (2012) work on trajectories and types of loss. The chapter discussed the progressive, ambiguous, and acknowledged forms of loss in relation to the advancing ageing of an older parent at the end of life. I highlight how this can result in a detachment from some of the emotional bonds with a loved one in order to psychologically defend against the devastation of the final loss. I also indicated the ways in which those psychological connections may be rebuilt through a process of continuing bonds, which may include spiritual dimensions, an internalised relationship with the loved one, or through legacy creation tasks. Difficult, or dysfunctional, relationships with parents can complicate this grief process.

The order of parental death can also have important consequences for the way the loss is grieved, and the impact it has on the adult child. The death of the first parent can sometimes see the grief subsumed into the grief of a remaining parent. Yet the death of a second parent can leave an adult child feeling 'orphaned'. In both losses there may be a change in role and responsibilities for the adult child. They may be expected to take on caring tasks for a first remaining parent or take on a position of family responsibility following the death of the second parent. Finally, there is a recognition that the adult child is in a period of mid- to late midlife which is often a period of awakening in terms of mortality awareness. This can create a sense of urgency for personal fulfilment and a feeling that there is only a window of opportunity to 'get things done'. Caring for, and/or managing a loss of, a parent in later life can impact upon this, increasing the sense of urgency due to the generational shift, yet finding fulfilment, reciprocity, and pleasure in the caring role, but also, for some, feeling that care is a burden which disrupts this period.

Limitations of the study

There are notable limitations with this study, and I invite further research into these areas. First, the original sample was entirely White British. I recognise that different cultures and religions will have different caregiving experiences, motives, expectations, family arrangements, and different ways of managing loss. Having completed a previous project into the role of faith and how those in midlife cope with heightened mortality awareness, I recognised the complexity of intersectionality on this topic. The geographical area of my research was predominantly White British, so this is where I chose to place my focus. Although there was some diversity with regards to class, this again is another area which requires further investigation. However, I predict comparable issues with regards to making decisions of care, how possessions are dealt with, and how losses are managed. It would also be interesting for future research to explore how sibling coordination can be mapped onto different socioeconomic backgrounds and how equity amongst siblings is perceived.

Another limitation is that the book is primarily focused upon a traditional structure of the family, and this is due to two reasons. One is that all the participants who responded to the invitation to be interviewed just so happened to have a traditional family structure of mother, father, and child/ren (some adult children had step-parents and one was adopted, but these relationships were not a key focus in the interviews). I did not deliberately seek out other permutations of family arrangements. I acknowledge that there may be some differences, as well as possible similarities, with the caregiving relationship and loss of a step-parent or someone else who has taken on that parental role for the child – such as a foster carer, friend, adoptive parent, other close family member, or mentor. Deliberately sampling these different family arrangements would have overcomplicated the current project, but more work is welcomed in this area.

Longitudinal research would also be interesting on this topic, following the phases and changes in dealing with the loss of older parents. I can envisage important future work which follows complete family groups, and I can see research of this kind creating case studies with the siblings and parents over a period of time as they navigate this journey into later life.

Finally, a limitation to this book is in its consideration of the traumatic impact of COVID-19. The pandemic saw an enormous impact on the way care services were run. There was a loss of support services in the community which family caregivers relied upon. Visits were restricted to the home and often staff had to think of inventive ways to facilitate relationships, including increasing the use of technology to contact relatives, and window visits. Access to medical care was affected due to the scaling back of provision by services within the NHS, with increased wait times, and the migration to the use of online platforms and telephone-based support which was not always suitable for those of advancing age. In-home care provision was also impacted because of the risk to paid caregivers and risk to the older person in receipt of care. This meant that adult children, who had previously relied upon paid caregivers, were thrust once again, and unexpectedly, into that caregiving role.

Future thinking about the child–parent caregiver relationship

I have illustrated in this book that there is a significant impact, physically and mentally, on the midlife adult child when caring for an older parent. Increased stress levels following a period of intensive caring, or the loss of a parent, can result in greater physical problems, result in unhealthy coping mechanisms, and increase morbidity amongst adult children. Parental loss in later life is also associated with poorer psychological well-being in comparison to those who have both parents still alive (Marks et al, 2007, p 1628). It is hoped that this book will increase awareness, for health-care professionals, care home staff, psychologists and therapists, and educators, of psychologically and physically demanding nature caring for a parent has on adult children. Often the focus is on the experiences of the older person, and, in this process, the adult child is the 'forgotten client' (Pratt et al, 1987).

My findings suggest that family members may have different needs and experiences throughout the parental-caregiving experience. Support programmes would be welcome in helping adult children manage the gradual and ambiguous loss of their parent, to understand the grieving process, and to understand how acutely this loss can be felt even before their parent's final death. Education programmes would be welcome in understanding the conditions such as dementia, or on types of loss, and how to navigate the care system. There is also a need for health-care professionals to help facilitate conversations around decision-making and to impartially set out the available options. More joined-up support from services to assist with housing, tax advice, power of attorney, and financial advice would be welcomed by adult children. The system of financial and legal issues to be arranged during this time can feel overwhelming, so a single point of support is important.

Schemes such as those run by My Home Life England show great initiative in bridging intergenerational divides and divides between care homes and the outside world. These community links are vital in being able to help facilitate relationships within care homes and with external resources and connections. Connections, like the community visitors, enable care staff to carry out more instrumental care tasks and at the same time the presence of volunteers helps facilitate experiences which enhance older peoples' well-being. Following the principle of appreciative enquiry there is a need to move away from intrusive governance, stifling and restrictive risk-adverse practice and the blame culture on care homes, to instead recognise the things that are working well, and helping care homes to support these good practices to happen more of the time.

Openness in talking about the challenges facing adult children and encouraging them to talk to their parents about future care plans is also important. Having courageous discussions about care and future death can ensure that the older parent's wishes are respected, and if these are communicated across the family then this could mean fewer family conflicts when crucial decisions have to be made. Similarly, if lasting power of attorney is established in advance, wills are prepared, there is a clear designation of roles and responsibilities, and paperwork is organised, then this can relieve the adult child of significant stress as they navigate their way through this experience.

The transition from a personal home to residential care can be a traumatic experience for older people and their families, the impact of which should not be underestimated. A move to care happens for two key reasons: when there is a change in the health status of the older person and when there is a change in the ability of the adult child to be able to care for them. Admission into a care home can feel overwhelming and frightening. It is important for carers to recognise that although the pre-admission process and meeting might be an everyday occurrence for them, for the older person moving into care this is a major life event. It is also important to carefully consider the emotions of the adult child, feelings of grief, loss, relief, anxiety, and fear are all heightened, which can impact on the way the adult child relates to their parent and to the care home staff. Encouraging a continuity of care, understanding individual needs, and having caring conversations with adult children is equally as important in this pre-admission phase to ensure a positive transition to care for their parents.

Final thoughts

Through navigating the emotional landscape of the child–parent caregiving experience I have revealed the complex practical, psychological, and emotional nature of the task. I have argued that the support of adult children to care for older parents, whether at home or by continuing their role to some extent within a care setting, is the cornerstone to older adult social care.

I hope that by raising awareness of the nuanced psychological challenges that adult child caregivers face, and through education and information, through genuine care and emotional support, we will improve the lives of those in the midlife generations and those that they provide care for. By social care providers enabling a more active, participatory, and supportive role for adult childen, visiting parents in a care home can become enjoyable and give the adult child the confidence to know that their relationship, although changed, can still flourish and be fulfilling.

Researching the child–parent caregiving relationship

The empirical research upon which this book is based was grounded in a psychosocial methodological approach, which examines the psychical processes that accompany socio-level experiences and brings a unique, multileveled understanding to the study of ageing, intergenerational relationships, and the life course. A psychosocial approach draws on insights, techniques, and theory from both psychoanalysis and sociology in order to understand the relationship between individual subjectivity and the social world. It recognises that there are psychical conflicting forces and tensions which exist between the internal world of the individual and the external, social world.

There has been a growing interest and significant expansion over the last twenty years in the area of psychosocial studies on a national and international level. Important studies in the psychosocial field have included explorations of love (Brown, 2006), intimacy, friendship, and transgenerational identification (Roseneil, 2006, 2009), and the fear of crime (Hollway and Jefferson, 2000), but so far there have been no identified studies that have used this approach to understand the subjective experiences of ageing and intergenerational relationships in later life.

An observance of the psychological dynamics of the research encounter with my participants played a vital role in developing a greater understanding of the experiences of ageing and intergenerational relationships in later life. For instance, in the initial stages of the research, I discovered, through a process of free association analysis, that taboo thoughts and ambiguous feelings about older parents were being expressed, feelings such as relief and liberation following the death of a parent, or once a parent had moved into care. These socially unacceptable attitudes are not always easily expressed through words, but through a psychosocial exploration these feelings could be revealed.

The projects

This book brings together the empirical and theoretical findings from four empirical projects and three systematic literature reviews which have been carried out over the last 16 years (2006–2022). The first empirical project entitled 'The Negotiation of Midlife: Exploring the Subjective Experience of Ageing' (2011), looked at the experience of men and women in the midlife phase of the life course with particular focus on the intergeneration relationships between adult children and their ageing parents. The two projects which followed were separate evaluations of two related projects run by My Home Life Essex Community Association. The first was an evaluation of a community visitors scheme which followed the experiences of volunteers who were recruited to go into care homes in Essex in order to build connections with older residents. The volunteer's task was relatively undefined, leaving freedom of expression as to how their role might take shape. The second project was an evaluation of My Home Life England – Friends and Neighbours (FaNs), which is a scheme to 'promote and support community engagement' between local care homes and their surrounding communities in order to unlock a range of resources and 'enrich the lives of care home residents'. Volunteers from the previous evaluation were key to building connections with the local community. One FaNs campaign involved wish-granting for residents, in which older people were asked what they wished for. These wishes were then pinned to a 'wishing washing line' in public places such as local supermarkets and were replicated on social media, The public could then offer to grant the wish and FaNs would coordinate the wish-granting. Other FaNs campaigns involved building intergenerational connections between local schools, the university, youth organisations, and local care homes.

I conducted these two evaluations with my colleague Chris Tanner (University of Essex). The combined fieldwork for these two evaluations involved mapping care home provision across Essex (UK); analysing a database of all care homes in Essex which recorded initial engagement with the FaNs scheme; and conducting a series of in-depth qualitative interviews with a range of professionals involved in the care provision for older people, including a total of ten care home managers, twelve interviews with the community visitor volunteers (CVs), one interview with a care home activities coordinator, and five interviews with other My Home Life England members. In addition, we conducted three focus groups, each with six care home staff, and carried out thirteen systematic psychosocial observations in eight care homes across the East of England. We also conducted in-depth qualitative interviews with care home residents and adult child relatives in each of the homes. Primarily we were interviewing about the impact these schemes made upon the lives of older people living in care, but I combined the interviews with the additional research agenda of exploring life in care more generally. I was aware that, as a researcher, I had an ethical duty to not over-research the same population of 'at-risk' participants. I did not want to have to return to the same care homes and the same willing residents in order to conduct research for my own separate research goals. As there was an overlap in the research agendas, I used the evaluation research as an opportunity to explore the stories of older people for a dual purpose.

Chris Tanner and I, as part of the evaluations, explored documentary evidence on the impact of the schemes by looking reflective diaries collected from the volunteers. We also regularly attended and observed the six-weekly community visitor meetings, which were designed to support and develop the volunteers. The community visitor's project received ethical approval from the University of Essex's ethics committee and the FaNs project received ethical approval from the University of Essex and the University of East London's research ethics committees. Both applications were submitted with the awareness of the dual purpose of the research aims.

In addition to the empirical data collected in these three major empirical projects this book draws upon a substantial and systematic scoping literature review on 'midlife orphans' which I carried out in collaboration with colleagues from the Open University: Rosalind Barbour, Michael Barbour, and Carol Komaromy. We conducted a search of the databases, ASSIA, Social Sciences Citation Index, PsychInfo, Social Policy, Medline, and CINAHL. We identified 113 suitable articles, on the themes of 'adults and parental death' (30 articles), 'bereavement in adult life' (8 articles), 'bereavement in older people' (30 articles), 'relatives/carers' experiences' (32 articles), 'the elderly' (6 articles) and 'bereavement care' (7 articles). As a team we read through all of these articles and identified key themes around the social discourses concerning the death of parents and the psychological impact of the loss. These co-researchers later published *Narratives of Parental Death, Dying, and Bereavement* (Pearce and Komaromy, 2021) based upon some of these findings.

In 2015 I was awarded funding and ethical approval from the University of East London to bring the data from all these projects together under an umbrella project I called 'The Impossible Choice?: Making Decisions of Care for and with Older Parents', and to fund the creation of a new empirical data set to supplement these existing data sets. This umbrella project created an addition of ten in-depth interviews with adult child relatives (aged 45–68) who had to make decisions of care for an older parent; four more interviews with community visitor volunteers; four additional interviews with care home managers; eleven additional interviews with older people (aged between 79 and 100) in residential care in two care homes in Essex; and an updated systematic literature review of an additional 110 articles on caring for older parents and the loss of older parents. I conducted a further systematic literature review in 2022 to update the literature, reading a further 72 articles, particularly around the issues of COVID-19 and the crisis in care. Table A1.1 shows the breakdown of the data collection process across the different projects.

Sadly, there is not the space to include every contributor's story in this book, but they all helped form a greater picture of the relationships between

Table A1.1: Outline of projects

	The Negotiation of Midlife: Exploring the Subjective Experience of Ageing (2005–2011)	The Midlife Orphan' Systematic Literature Review (2013)	My Home Life Essex Community Visitor Scheme Evaluation (2013–2014) (Morgan Brett and Tanner, 2014)	Care Home Friends and Neighbours Evaluation (2016–2017) (Morgan Brett and Tanner, 2017)	The Impossible Choice? Making Decisions of Care for and with Older Parents (2014–2015)
	The University of Essex	The Open University	The University of Essex	The University of Essex; The University of East London	The University of East London
	Bethany Morgan Brett	Bethany Morgan Brett; Rosaline S. Barbour; Carol Komaromy; Michael Barbour	Bethany Morgan Brett; Chris Tanner	Bethany Morgan Brett; Chris Tanner	Bethany Morgan Brett
	ESRC Scholarship PhD data		Joseph Rowntree funded		Early career accelerator grant
				The University of Essex and the University of East London's ethics committees in 2015	
	45 psychosocial interviews with 22 men and women aged 40–60	113 articles	7 observations of care homes; 1 observation of MHLECA/home managers meeting; 9 interviews and discussions with older people; 12 interviews with community visitors; 5 observations of community visitor meetings; 5 interviews with care home managers; 3 interviews with MHLECA staff; 1 interview with Essex QI lead; 3 focus groups with 6 staff in each care home; 3 interviews with friends and relatives of older people	7 interviews with care home managers and staff; 4 interviews with FaNs volunteers or contributing organisations; 1 interview with local FaNs coordinator; 2 interviews with MHLECA members; 7 interviews with older people in care homes; 2 observations in different care homes; Attendance at conferences and meetings organised by MHLECA	10 interviews with adult child relatives (aged 45–70); 4 interviews with community visitors; 3 interviews with care home managers; 11 interviews with care home residents; 110 articles for literature review Updated literature review of 72 articles in 2022
					Total data collection 127 interviews; 9 care home observations; 3 focus groups; 5 observations of meetings; 295 journal articles

adult children and their older parents. A list of the participants mentioned in this book are included in Appendix 2, Tables A2.1–A2.3.

Researching 'at-risk' groups

Carrying out social research with care home residents requires the careful balance of protecting vulnerable older people, whilst also making sure that the research is inclusive and hears the voices of a typically marginalised population. Ethics committees are understandably cautious about approving care home research, as I found when it took 8 months (out of the 12-month FaNs project) to gain approval from the very committee I was a senior member of.

By very definition, care home residents will have some level of vulnerability or are considered 'at risk'. An older person may be considered at risk because they are less able to protect themselves from harm, abuse, or exploitation. The UK's Office of the Public Guardian safeguarding policy (section 5.2) has moved away from the term 'vulnerable' as it implies that some of the fault for the abuse could lie with the victim of abuse and instead uses the term 'at risk' to refer to these populations (Morgan Brett and Wheeler, 2022; Office of the Public Guardian safeguarding policy, 2023). But just because someone is considered 'at risk' does not mean that they are at risk of an immediate danger. For older people in care, their 'risk' may be a result of a mental or physical impairment or arise from their social environment (in this case the dependency that they have on the home and the staff within that home). It is important to balance out the duty to protect those at risk with the right to participate (Morgan Brett and Wheeler, 2022). By assuming that a particular group of individuals, such as those living in care homes, are incapable of making the decision to participate in social research can deprive them of the right to have their opinions heard. Yet there remains a balancing act of promoting the benefits of participation for older people with the risks that might be involved. Being interviewed and participating in research can be empowering for some people, as they get to tell their side of a story which might get missed in official or more dominant forms of discourse. Researchers should not be unnecessarily protective and make assumptions about the ability of people to make rational decisions that are in their own best interests. Respondents should have the option to refuse or withdraw participation in research and, if they feel fully informed about the research, they should have the right to participate, as long as there is no risk of harm.

Working within the Mental Capacity Act

Although many of the older people who live in care homes have the capacity to understand and contribute in an informed way to the research being carried out, others may be classed as more at risk than others and may be seen to lack the mental capacity to understand what is being asked of them. Defining the level of 'mental capacity' of a resident can be difficult and, indeed, as a social researcher (or even through my experience as a psychotherapist), I do not have the medical knowledge to make a judgement about the capacity of any resident to give consent, and to *assume* a lack of capacity can be demeaning and unethical. Dobson (2008, p 4) states 'researchers should assume that a participant or potential participant does have the capacity to decide whether to consent or not to their participation, unless there is evidence that questions the person's capacity to reach this decision'. I therefore found it an important part of the recruitment process to involve senior staff in care homes to help identify residents who would be best able to assist with the research. However, this was less than ideal in terms of developing a representative sample of residents. Staff naturally tended to recommend the chattiest, liveliest, friendliest, and most content residents who were most able (or likely) to give a more positive account of life in the care home. After one interview with a resident, the manager asked, "I take it no one said anything bad then about the home?" Even now I am still unsure as to how to get around this dilemma in care home research, but I think being aware of this dynamic and reflecting upon its impact is an important part of the research.

Another thing to consider is that the mental functioning of older people, particularly in early dementia, can be progressive or variable. I found that there was the potential for an older person to understand and contribute in a lucid way to start with in an interview, but this state could change if they became unwell, tired, or stressed in any way. As a researcher it was important for me to be aware of changes in cognition and draw an interview to a close and inform a member of staff if there were concerns. The Mental Capacity Act defines this protocol:

> During the course of conducting a project, researchers may become aware that participants who initially had given valid consent have lost that capability in later stages of the project. In order legally to conduct the research, the usual research process would need to be halted, the protocol revised and ethical opinion re-sought before non-consenting participants could again participate (MCA, Section 34 (2)). (Dobson, 2008, p 9)

For a resident to have the 'mental capacity' to consent means that a participant needs to understand that you are conducting a 'study' or piece of 'research' which will result in a 'report' or other 'research outputs' (book, website, presentations, articles, and so on). They need to understand that they are being asked to 'talk about their experience or give their opinion', and they can say 'no' or 'stop at any time', and 'that this will not result in any detriment to them or the care that they receive'. It is important to phrase this information in an easy to understand yet informative manner, which is also delivered in a non-patronising way. Some residents may have previous experience of conducting research themselves in earlier years or may have taken part in other research projects, so may be very familiar with the research language, whereas others may not know key words such as 'research outputs' or 'informed consent' or 'withdrawal', so this will need explaining clearly and concisely.

Of course, research with individuals who do not have the mental capacity to give informed consent is possible but involves a more rigorous and external ethical process than can be approved at a university-level research committee. Applications for research with this group of participants should be approved by the NHS Health Research Authority's Social Care Research Ethics Committee, and for short, small-scale research this is not always a feasible option. As such, my research ethics applications for the 'FaNs Evaluation' and 'The Impossible Choice?' projects were approved by the University of East London's Ethics Committee (UREC) and I decided to not include any adults who the staff assessed to not have the mental capacity to give consent to participate. I also did not interview others (such as carers or relatives) as proxy respondents, as the legal position in England and Wales is that where adults lack the capacity to consent, no other person can be authorised to give proxy consent according to the Mental Capacity Act (Dobson, 2008, p 10).

Gaining informed consent

As in all social science research, informed consent to participate forms an important and underlying ethical principle. In all interviews with care home residents, I sought informed consent before proceeding with any recorded interview and ideally this was in a written form. I designed a simple consent form with a series of boxes to be ticked, which divided the different elements of the research that they were consenting too. In instances where I deemed written consent to be inappropriate or hindering the research process in some way, I read through the consent form with the resident, recording this conversation and the agreements that they made in the research. In line with the Mental Capacity Act, I did not ask for consent from anyone (for example staff or relative) on behalf of the older person. If a resident could not or did not want to consent, I did not include them.

During the process of recruitment of participants, I distributed information sheets in the form of a printed leaflet, which outlined who I was, what the research was about, and what might be expected of them should they choose to contribute. These were given out approximately one week before I returned to go through the consent form and check their understanding of the project. Providing timely information about the research and what I was asking them to consent to gave my participants time to think about whether they were still happy to take part. Included in any ethical procedure in social research is the right to withdraw, so during this week's gap my participants could make a clear, thoughtful decision about participation, and I also reminded them that they could withdraw during or immediately after the research should they wish.

All participants signed and dated a consent form which stated that they understood the nature of the research, what their participation would involve, how to withdraw from the research, and what their data would be used for and how it would be stored. With regards to anonymisation, the strategy was different across the projects. In 'The Negotiation of Midlife' project all participants were anonymised, however I recognised in the later evaluations and in 'The Impossible Choice?' project the importance of offering the control over anonymisation to the participant. This is particularly important when researching at-risk populations. Clark (2013, p 71) writes that 'anonymising respondents also serves to hide, marginalise or silence the voices of groups and individuals for whom engaging in research may be intended to be an emancipatory experience'. As such, I offered participants from all sample sets the opportunity to use their real name, choose a pseudonym for themselves, or allow me to choose one for them. Most opted for me to choose a pseudonym for them. Some initially chose to use their real name, but then decided that the stories they had told me were too sensitive and changed them. Some kept their real names, and some chose a name for themselves. However, throughout this book I have deliberately used names of participants without distinguishing which names were real and which were not. Care homes have also not been identified by their real names. They have also not been specifically geographically identified; however, it can be known that the care homes in which the research was carried out were based in Essex, in the East of England, and some of the care homes mentioned by adult child participants were based in areas around North London.

Adult child: sampling

The adult child caregivers represented in this book were all aged between 39 and 68 years old. In the project 'The Negotiation of Midlife' (2011) I interviewed twenty-two British born men and women, aged 39–57 years old, who – all but one – had children. I interviewed this sample on at least two occasions each. The ten adult child relatives interviewed for 'The Impossible Choice?' project were aged between 45 and 68 and six of these ten participants had children. I selected the majority of my sample groups for both projects through a convenience and snowball sampling method. The sample included a range of socio-economic backgrounds, and a diverse range of experiences of caring for older parents, from having a parent who was fit and well but where discussions of future care had arisen, to those who had made the decision for their parent to go into institutional care, to those whose parents had subsequently died.

Ethnicity

I chose to *not* include an ethnically and culturally diverse sample and all participants identified as White British except one British-born Black woman, 'Jeanette', interviewed for 'The Negotiation of Midlife' project. The first rationale for the narrow ethnic sample is that the two key geographical areas from which most of the participants were sampled had a predominantly White British population (83 per cent in the East of England and 66 per cent in the North London borough (Office for National Statistics, 2019), which I will keep anonymous). In researching care homes across Essex, I noticed that older people in care homes were much less likely to be from ethnically diverse populations, indeed I did not meet a single older person from an ethnic minority; every care home resident was White British. The second reason that the sample was not ethnically diverse was this would have significantly changed the focus of the projects. In a much earlier research project in 2004 I explored the death of parents and its effect on the midlife adult through the lens of two religious perspectives, Christianity and Buddhism. From this early research, and from supervising other research projects which focused on the experiences of families from ethnic minorities caring for parents, and from subsequent reading around this topic, I identified the vast complexity of looking at care decisions through diverse cultural and religious perspectives. Each minority (religious or cultural) group has a very different set of specific needs (cultural, language, dietary, or religious) which can affect their health seeking behaviour and care decisions. Ethnic and racial diversity in caregiving practices, and their associated generational differences, has significant implications for the study of caring for older parents and for social policy for health-care providers. There can be specific cultural expectations around caring for parents such as loyalty and filial responsibility. For example, in traditional Chinese culture, 'adult children are expected to care for their aging parents, contribute financially, and provide emotional support (Weng & Nguyen, 2011)' (Miyawaki, 2020). And there is an expression of obligation and expectation in caregiving practices in cultures in the Global South, for example in Nepal, a 'reciprocal exchange of care between the parents and children was associated with the religious conception of virtue and vice' (Raut, 2018, p 288). Caring for older parents is built into the systems of family life in many traditional societies. Extended families might live together in intergenerational systems of care. This is common in some African countries, such as Nigeria where there can be a sense of indebtedness to older parents for the care provided when the adult child was younger: 'Generally, adult children perceived the need to reciprocate past support received from their older parents' (Akinrolie et al, 2020, p 478). In Western cultures, such as that of the United Kingdom, families are more likely to live in geographically dispersed regions and less likely to live together in the family home. This is, not least, because British homes are not always designed with an extended family in mind and accommodating an older parent might take significant adaptations and/or extensions to a property in order for them to move in.

The Care Quality Commission recognises that ethnic minority groups often feel that their cultural needs are not met in care home settings and resultantly are more likely to be cared for by family at home (CQC, 2016). As such, the ethnic minorities are vastly unrepresented in UK care homes (certainly in the East of England). The NHS Digital reported that the percentage of adults receiving long-term support in care homes who were White was 83.3 per cent in 2021, down from 87.8 per cent in 2016. This book therefore focuses on the experiences of the White British-born population, with the acknowledgement that this is a limitation of this book, and more research needs to be done to explore these stories in more detail.

Transcription

Interviews across all the projects were audio recorded and a single interview ranged anywhere from 20 minutes to 4 hours in length. The adult children relatives in my PhD were interviewed twice, and one participant was interviewed on three occasions, and these lasted between 2 and 3 hours per interview (totalling 4–6 hours with each participant). In 'The Impossible Choice?' project, adult child relatives were interviewed for around 3–4 hours. Across all projects each interview was transcribed using verbatim transcription protocols. I transcribed around half of the data myself, but the other half was transcribed by professional transcribers. All transcripts were initially annotated in a 'free association' analysis, exploring the initial emotional response to the data, and thinking of 'what comes to mind' when reading it. All field notes were also transcribed, which was also able to capture some of the non-verbal, visual communication which took place in the encounters, but which the audio-recording was unable to record. The analytical approach is described later in this chapter.

Methodological approaches
Researching adult children: a psychosocial approach

In researching adult child relatives of older parents I wanted to get a detailed sense of the emotional impact witnessing the ageing of parents has upon them. I wanted to understand the complex inner psychic conflicts which are evoked by the experience of personal ageing and witnessing the ageing of another, but which are not necessarily expressed directly through language. I wanted to explore the emotional lives of my interviewees. My interest lay in the specific social experiences and cultural expectations which influence my interviewee's attitudes and pragmatic reactions to ageing and how this is intertwined with the unconscious psychic processes, conflicts, and ambivalences that they experienced in their inner emotional worlds. I argue that our conscious narratives are screened by our unconscious and mediated by social norms. A psychosocial approach (Hollway and Jefferson, 2000; Roseneil, 2006) seeks to access motivations, drives, and impulses which operate at an unconscious level.

As a psychosocial researcher and psychotherapist, I am interested in the material held in the unconscious part of the psyche. We might visualise the unconscious as a treasure chest of information about the individual's psychology, consisting of impulsive urges, primitive drives, and deep-rooted anxieties, all of which our psyches would rather keep psychologically contained there. Our minds employ a number of psychological tactics called ego-defences in order to keep these destructive and demanding impulses under control (Freud, 1992 [1936]). These ego-defences operate at the level of the unconscious and they prevent the ego from becoming overwhelmed by denying or distorting the reality of the situation. Some of the ego-defences include (amongst others) denial, repression, regression, projection, and sublimation (Freud, 1992 [1936]). Moreover, unconscious material can be observed through parapraxes such as jokes, Freudian slips of the tongue or pen, or through unconscious body language, and through dreams (Freud and Strachey, 1965 [1900]). Psychosocial researchers are interested in accessing unconscious material in order to give a comprehensive understanding of the emotional experience of the individual they are observing. They are interested not only in the words spoken in a verbal, conscious way, but also in the emotional experience of the interview encounter. Hoggett argued that 'we communicate *affectively* as well as discursively and we do this precisely because of the inherent limitations of language in expressing experience' (2008, p 381, italics my own). Language is not always sufficient in understanding human emotional experience; some feelings are beyond words, and it is only through affectively feeling the emotion that some things can be truly understood.

In studying the child–parent caregiving relationship in later life, and its associated losses and other emotional challenges, I needed a method which would allow me access to deeper levels of emotional expression, admittance into the world of taboo thoughts, and a greater understanding of the primitive feelings and drives which happen at an unconscious level when thinking about parental relationships. In order to access this kind of material I used psychoanalytical techniques such as observing transference, countertransference, and projective identification in the interview encounter. I considered the slips in the narrative, the inconsistencies, and the silences. By employing a psychosocial approach, it enabled me to look beyond the words and wider discourse, and to understand unconscious motivations and emotions, and to reveal 'who we are' in relation with others (Parker, 2010).

A psychosocial method, as set out by Hollway and Jefferson (2000), adopts some techniques commonly employed in clinical psychoanalysis and applies them to the social research interview and its subsequent analysis. It pays close attention to emotions, thoughts, and motivations, and whereas some sociological interviews tend to acknowledge these features only at a conscious level, a psychosocial interviewer will also take into account unconscious dynamics and processes. The production of data in a psychosocial interview comes from the relationship between the interviewer and interviewee, both of whom come to the interview situation with their own anxieties, defences, and histories which can affect the material that is created in the interview. Hollway and Jefferson stated that in their research using this method they,

> intend to construe both the researcher and researched as anxious defended subjects, whose mental boundaries are porous where unconscious material is concerned. This means that both will be subject the projections and introjections of ideas and feelings coming from the other person. It also means that the impressions that we have about each other are not derived simply from the 'real' relationship, but that what we say and do in the interaction will be mediated by internal fantasies which derive from our histories of significant relationships. (2000, p 45)

I suggest that being aware of the unconscious processes at work in the interview can give the researcher a deeper insight into the motivations of the interviewee in the way that they construct their stories. I support the idea that in all interviews the interviewee is what Hollway and Jefferson call 'defended', and this is particularly true in interviews dealing with highly sensitive or emotional topics, such as the themes that I am interested in – that of intergenerational relationships, ageing, loss, disappointment, and death. I would argue, as Hollway and Jefferson have, that a defended subject may not tell you the full story, whether that is conscious or unconscious. Some things are too difficult to talk about or to express, often because they threaten to break down emotional defences. By becoming aware of the defences and the underlying reasons for these, an enriched understanding of the interviewees' deep-rooted feelings can be attained, enabling the interviewer to recognise the undercurrent of emotions which underpin the socially acceptable front that is performed on a much more conscious level. Every interviewee is necessarily psychically defended – everyone has an unconscious which contains motivations, instincts, and impulses which are constrained by the social world in which they live. In different social situations this struggle between the inner and outer world fluctuates, making the individual more or less defended depending on the circumstances.

For the project 'The Negotiation of Midlife' I used a psychosocial method as developed by Hollway and Jefferson (2000) in *Doing Qualitative Research Differently*, in which they suggested that the incorporation of psychoanalysis into social research methods required a very specific interview technique and new ways of analysing the information gathered. In their own research Hollway and Jefferson conducted two interviews with each interviewee. The first used a free association technique in a life story or biographical interview, keeping the questioning style as open as possible and letting the interviewee's ideas, views, and story emerge as much as possible in their own words. This free association method follows the direction of the interviewee's 'ordering and phrasing' of their story (Hollway and Jefferson, 2000, p 53). It also allowed the interviewer to look critically at any inconsistencies and contradictions, which could then be checked in the second interview through a series of narrative questions based upon the first interview. The second interview was an opportunity to ask some more structured questions in order to make some comparisons between interviewees. It involved asking 'tailor-made' questions based on issues which seemed to cause the conflicts in the narrative. The interviewing process was then followed by a detailed analysis of the experience as a whole, including the relationship between the interviewee and the interviewer, the emotions involved, examining the words in the transcript and a careful consideration of the narrative construction.

Like Hollway and Jefferson, I conducted two interviews with each interviewee and on one occasion I conducted three interviews. I originally aimed for the interviews to be one week apart but due to practical and geographical constraints this was not always possible and the gap between was sometimes up to a couple of months. This method of double interviewing my participants was a valuable one as it enabled me to explore some of the psychodynamics of the first interview and to take into consideration this in the second interview. I was able to follow up on leads, hunches, and ideas which arose in the first interview. The first interview was more open-ended than the second. Although I took inspiration from Hollway and Jefferson's method of interviewing, I did not follow it rigidly. A free association method requires a certain amount of courage, and it is too easy to revert to the security of the interview schedule and its predefined questions. In the initial stages of interviewing there was the constant worry and danger that without this safety net the conversation would dry up and I would not know how to develop a certain lead. It took a few attempts with my own interviewees to relinquish some of this control over the interviews, and although I asked some questions I tried as far as possible in my later interviews to allow the interviewees' narratives to develop according to their own direction of thought.

During the interview I took mental notes about my interviewees' body language, verbal and bodily expression, the use of the physical space, demeanour, and presentation of self, which I then wrote down immediately after the interviews. I also kept a comprehensive record of my own impressions and feelings about each interview. A psychosocial approach requires critical reflection by the interviewer in order to monitor the process. The psychosocial interviewer needs to be constantly questioning: 'Why has this person said this?', 'Why at this moment?', and, just as importantly, 'Why did I respond in this way and how did it reflect the interview?' (Roper, 2003, p 27). This is where the issues of transference and countertransference come into play. The psychosocial interviewer needs to be constantly questioning their reflexivity, asking: 'Why did they make me feel like that?', 'How did I deal with it?', and 'How did that affect the interview?' Frosh and Baraitser (2008, p 359) described reflexivity as requiring the researcher to:

> keep an honest gaze on what s/he brings to the research process: how s/he sets it up, what is communicated to the subject, what differences of race, class, gender etc might prevail and what impact they might have, and how her/his actions might influence the subject's own active meaning–making activities.

Both interviewer and interviewee necessarily bring their own personal and emotional biographies into the interview encounter and they will form impressions about each other based upon these backgrounds. However, these positions are not fixed and are constantly adapting throughout the encounter. It is the exploration of these dynamics which can be a valuable technique for supplementing the analysis.

Researching older parents: a phenomenological approach

With the sample of care home residents, I was aware at how physically and emotionally taxing a psychosocial interview might be for them, particularly given the length of the interviews. Some residents were hard of hearing, some visually impaired, others generally quite tired. I decided to still use an in–depth qualitative interview approach, but more through the lens of phenomenology. Interpretive phenomenology is rooted in the philosophy of Husserl (1954), which seeks to uncover the lived experience of others. In this approach the researcher puts aside preconceptions and prejudices so as not to bias the data collection. This method of data collection involves 'studying things in their natural settings, attempting to make sense of, or interpret, phenomena in terms of the meaning that people bring to them' (Denzin and

Lincoln, 2005, p 3). With this method, the researcher is able to get a sense of the lived experience of those experiencing it. Participants are given the freedom to describe the phenomenon of interest and to show the researcher what is of meaningful significance. In practice this allowed me to observe care home communal areas and speak to residents about their day-to-day lives. It allowed for rich, in-depth interviews with residents, as well as being given a glimpse into their lives in care and their private spaces within the home. They sometimes showed me objects or photos which meant something to them: one lady demonstrated how well she could walk with her walking frame decorated with fairy lights, another showed me her finger-prick test for her blood sugar levels, some showed me photos of their family or of themselves in the past or talked to me about a prized or sentimental possession. These interviews were collaborative, conversational, and interactional, based on the assumption that all knowledge is co-constructed.

Researching care homes: an observational approach

In the 'Care Home Friends and Neighbours Evaluation' and 'The Community Visitor Evaluation', my colleague Chris Tanner and I conducted a series of observations in care homes, with permission of the care home managers. These observations were conducted solely in communal areas and not in personal spaces, although some general field notes relating to the interviews were taken in bedroom meetings too when relevant. The residents in these spaces knew that we were researchers and that we were observing the space. Chris Tanner and I took deliberately differing and complementary approaches to the ways in which we conducted these observations. Chris took a more psychoanalytic observational approach, taking the role of a complete observer (Gold, 1958), remaining detached from participatory activities. He did not take notes or make recordings in the settings but rather reflected internally on the feelings, emotions, and psychological dynamics of the group setting, recording detailed reflections immediately post-observation. I took a more participant-observer role (Gold, 1958), involving myself in tasks, activities, and conversations, and I recorded my notes in situ in a notebook and post-observations on a dictaphone which were later transcribed. I recorded feelings, thoughts, timings, the setting (including sketches of the layout of spaces), objects and physical effects in the space, people who came in and out of the space under observation, interactions between people, particularly with the residents, and events and activities within the space. Where I was carrying out short observations of the communal areas of the care homes, I did not formally observe residents who were considered not to have the mental capacity to consent, nor record any incidental observations with these individuals. However, as a guest in the resident's home, I behaved with courtesy and reciprocity if they engaged me in conversation. Chris Tanner and I compared each other's observations and provided one another with a 'critical eye' over which to analyse the differing viewpoints on the same setting. We also worked closely with a small committee of academics who formed an advisory group to share ideas and findings with.

Data analysis

Each discrete data set was initially analysed within its own research context. In 'The Negotiation of Midlife' project, I transcribed all the interviews in full and, in addition, I closely examined the emotional experience of the interview at the time and explored my emotional reactions to the data post-interview. I propose one of the key principles of psychosocial research is a full immersion into the data, that is, getting 'under the skin' of your interviewee and analysing the smallest gestures or moments of countertransference. Countertransference can be considered very simply as an indicator as to what is experienced in the mind of the other and is recognised through self-reflection and observation of one's own feelings. As Hollway and Jefferson said in their analytic process, they felt 'inhabited by that person in the sense that our imagination was full of him or her' (2000, p 69). I, too, found myself in that position, often thinking of, and dreaming about, my participants. I listened back to the audio recordings, allowing myself to become re-immersed in the interviewees' stories and feelings. I made self-reflexive notes during this process of revisiting the transcripts asking, 'How did I feel at particular points in the interview?' and 'How do I feel now when looking back over it?' I also read over the post-interview field observation notes to situate myself back in that experience.

By the time I had read through all my transcribed interviews, the amount of information I had gathered felt overwhelming. Hollway and Jefferson discuss the principle of Gestalt, stating that it 'is based on the idea that the whole is greater than the sum of the parts' and that 'we can appreciate better the Gestalt principle if it is understood also as the internal capacity for holding those data together in the mind' (2000, p 69). At this stage it was tempting to revert to qualitative computer software to help cope with all the information that needed to be systematically organised. Hollway and Jefferson warn against such analytic procedures as they feel that the fragmentation of data means that the complete picture is often lost (2000, p 69) They warn that a qualitative data program 'offers increasingly sophisticated ways of not holding the data as a whole in the mind, precisely as it affords ways of holding it outside of the mind' (2000, pp 68–9). I did use a qualitative data analysis package (MAXQDA), which I think was an indication of the early anxiety I felt about the overwhelming nature of the data. The process of using a computer-assisted qualitative data analysis software (CAQDAS) package such as MAXQDA involved uploading the interview transcripts, reading through them, and identifying themes in the data. These chunks of data were then extracted, coded, and analysed. Whereas an entire analysis could be based on this process, I used the system very sparingly to code people according to where they were in the life cycle and to look at patterns in the biographical situations of my interviewees. Instead, the majority of my data analysis was done through a process of free association on the transcripts. This involved having a transcript in front of me, immersing myself back into the situation of the interview, reflecting upon the feelings that were evoked and also reflecting on what I am reminded of when I am reading through the data – no matter how strange! (Please take a look at my SAGE case study, 'Uncovering the unconscious in psychosocial research' (Morgan Brett, 2018), for examples of transference and countertransference in the interviews.)

I was mindful of fragmenting my data and losing sight of the interview as a whole. I did not want to lose the subtleties between the links within the interviews nor did I want to lose to emotional experience of the interview which formed the very basis of a psychosocial approach. The basic coding and categorisation of my data proved useful, but I was also careful to re-examine and re-focus my analysis back on to the interviews as a whole once this initial coding was completed. Moreover, I learnt to trust myself to be able to hold and contain my interviewees' stories in a more 'affective' way. Their stories and emotional transferences had already been experienced by me and were already in my mind; it was just about me trusting myself to cope with this initially overwhelming experience.

In the two evaluations, Chris and I transcribed the entire data set of interviews, observation notes, and meeting notes, with the assistance of a professional transcriber. We conducted a free association analysis on the data and conducted a thematic analysis using MAXQDA. Thematic analysis is one of the most used methods for analysing qualitative interview data (Braun and Clarke, 2006, 2013; Rubin and Rubin, 2012; Spencer et al, 2014; King et al, 2019). Put simply, this approach involves systematically and closely reading all the data to find and label the recurring and distinctive features of the participants accounts, referred to as 'themes' (Morgan Brett and Wheeler, 2022). In these evaluations we were primarily exploring the themes relating to assessment of the two schemes, including how they were established, the impact they had on the lives of older people, the volunteers, and the culture of the care home. However, the dual nature of the research meant that I also analysed themes relating to life in the care home and the experience of transitioning to care.

The literature dataset for 'The Midlife Orphan project' was analysed using a framework analysis (Ritchie and Spencer, 1994). Ritchie and Spencer (1994) outline five stages to framework analysis: familiarisation; identifying a framework; indexing; charting; and mapping and interpretation. First we immersed ourselves in the reading of the data, getting an overall sense of, and developing an appraisal of, the existing literature on the death of parents in midlife. Next we identified a framework of codes which were emerging from the data (an inductive approach) and combined this with our initial a priori themes (a deductive approach). The next step involved an indexing of the data to organise the literature into our framework categories. We were then able to map the literature and draw some conclusions on the data set.

Finally, 'The Impossible Choice?: Making Decisions of Care for and with Older Parents', was an umbrella project which sought to integrate all the aforementioned projects, as well as creating a small new dataset to supplement and bring together the emerging thematic strands. This project involved an in-depth, thematic *re-analysis* of all the data I had collected across all the projects, with a new focus which would result in this book. For this I used the qualitative software NVivo, where I combined the all the collected primary data sets, already analysed literature, and added a new updated systematic literature review of another 110 articles on the death of parents, caring for older parents, ageing, and midlife.

Summary

This chapter has introduced the trajectory of research projects which have shaped and informed this book. It has outlined the practical and ethical challenges of conducting research for and with older people, and the importance of ensuring that this type of is empowering, inclusive, avoidant of exploitation, and gives voice to the older person. Careful consideration of situated ethics are important in this undertaking.

It has outlined a psychosocial approach (as set out by Hollway and Jefferson, 2000), and how this method has helped to reveal motivations, emotions, and feelings which are unconscious and are not always regulated or screened by the conscious self. It has been argued that psychosocial studies have begun to re-emerge in more recent scholarly practice and contemporary debates, perhaps as a conciliatory attempt to bridge the historical divide between the two disciplines of sociology and psychoanalysis. Borrowing psychoanalytic techniques and applying them in social research can help to illuminate another layer to the study of the human experience that sociology sometimes overlooks. Self-reflection and observance of transference and countertransference can become a means to free ourselves from the constraints imposed on our internal forces through repression and on our external forces through ideology (Habermas, 1968; Clarke, 2006). Furthermore, psychoanalysis can help uncover distortions and meanings in everyday language (Habermas, 1968; Clarke, 2006). These are important founding techniques in psychosocial studies, particularly as set out in Hollway and Jefferson's method, and have been particularly interesting and useful for understanding the often-unspoken, under-acknowledged, and stigmatised feelings of adult children.

APPENDIX 2

Participant charts

Table A2.1: Adult child participant biographical chart

Pseudonym	Age	Job	Marital status	Parental status	Siblings	Mum	Dad	Type and place of interview
Sharon	54	Works for a law firm; on a sabbatical	Single with partner	No children	One older sister	Aged 83 Living in a care home	Died from a heart attack aged 55	In-depth, psychosocial interview at participant's home
Fred	56	Civil engineer	Separated	Two teenage boys	One older brother	Died aged 85 from cancer	Died from dementia aged 88	In-depth, psychosocial interview at participant's home
Alison	63	Librarian	Married for 40 years	Three adult children – two boys and one girl; youngest adult child lives at home	One older sister	Died aged 97 from dementia	Dad died from bowel disease aged 87	In-depth, psychosocial interview at participant's home
Hazel	68	Researcher in health interventions	Single	No children	Only child	Mum died aged 100 from dementia	Dad died aged 79 from heart problems	In-depth, psychosocial interview at participant's home
Ruth	54	Charity worker	Same-sex partner	No children	Two brothers and a sister	Mum died aged 74 from vasculitis	Dad is in his 80s, has dementia and lives in care	In-depth, psychosocial interview at participant's home
Coleen	45	Legal secretary	Single	No children	Only child	Mum died from mental health problems aged 62	Dad is aged 74, has dementia, and lives in care	In-depth, psychosocial interview at participant's home
Teresa	55	Market Researcher	Married	4 children. All in 20s and 30s. All live independently	Two brothers and a sister	Mum died aged 78 from a heart attack	Dad lives independently abroad	In-depth, psychosocial interview at participant's home

Table A2.1: Adult child participant biographical chart (continued)

Pseudonym	Age	Job	Marital status	Parental status	Siblings	Mum	Dad	Type and place of interview
Patricia	55	Personal assistant and receptionist	Married	Three adult daughters, one who lives at home	One older sister and a brother who died in childhood	Mum died aged 80	Dad lives independently but needs some care	In-depth, psychosocial interview at participant's home
Lily	57	Life coach	Long-term partner	One daughter	Three siblings, and two half-siblings	Mum is aged 87 and lives in a care home; stepmother is aged 70 and lives independently	Dad died of a heart attack aged 70	In-depth, psychosocial interview held in a private space outside of the participant's home
Annie	70	Retired	Married	Has children – number unknown	One brother	Mum is aged 99, lives in care	Dad died – age and cause of death unknown	Convenient sampled, qualitative semi-structured interview in the care home
Jilly	68	Musician	Single	No children	One brother	Mum is aged 99 living in a care home	Dad – unknown; stepfather died aged 90	Convenient sampled, qualitative semi-structured interview in the care home
Trina	70	Retired	Long-term partner	Two daughters	One brother who lives abroad	Mum is aged 99 living in a care home (Diana)	Unknown	Convenient sampled, qualitative semi-structured interview in the care home

(continued)

Table A2.1: Adult child participant biographical chart (continued)

Pseudonym	Age	Job	Marital status	Parental status	Siblings	Mum	Dad	Type and place of interview
Rob	50	Computer technician	Divorced/ single	Two sons and a daughter; the two youngest children live with their mother	One younger sister	Mum is aged 79, lives at home but has dementia and requires care from Rob	Dad died from lung cancer aged 83	In-depth, psychosocial interview at participant's home
Jeff	48	Care worker	Single	No children	One sister who lives with their mother	Mum is aged 84, lives at home but requires extensive physical and emotional support from Jeff and his sister	Dad died from cancer when Jeff was a child	In-depth, psychosocial interview at participant's home
Angela	49	Self-employed business owner	Married	Two daughters – one teenager and one adult; both live at home	Only child	Mum is aged 74 and lives independently without care	Dad is aged 70 and lives independently without care	In-depth, psychosocial interview at participant's home
Sarah	39	Swimming teacher	Married	One young daughter and currently pregnant with second child	Two older brothers	Mum is aged 65 and lives independently without care	Dad is aged 70 and lives independently without care	In-depth, psychosocial interview at participant's home
Jeannette	45	Unemployed	Single	10-year-old twins	Only child	Adoptive mother died a few months before interview. Age unknown	Unknown – no relationship with biological father	In-depth, psychosocial interview at participant's home

Table A2.1: Adult child participant biographical chart (continued)

Pseudonym	Age	Job	Marital status	Parental status	Siblings	Mum	Dad	Type and place of interview
Joe	49	Management	Married	One adult son	One older brother and one older sister	Mum died in later life, age and cause of death unknown	Dad died aged 62 from lung disease	In-depth, psychosocial interview held in a private space outside of the participant's home
Matthew	55	Director	Married	Two adult children – son and a daughter	Three younger brothers	Mum is aged 79 and lives independently without care	Dad is aged 79 and lives independently without care	In-depth, psychosocial interview held in a private space outside of the participant's home
Diane	55	Care worker	Separated	Two adult daughters	Two younger sisters	Mum is aged 79 lives with Diane's sister and requires care	Dad died aged 64 from a stroke	In-depth, psychosocial interview at participant's home
Adrian	43	Technician	Divorced/ single	One young daughter who lives with her mum	One brother	Mum is aged 55 and lives independently without care	Dad is aged 67 and lives independently without care	In-depth, psychosocial interview held in a private space outside of the participant's home
Rodney	55	Unemployed	Married	Four adult children; a grandchild who lives with him	One brother and seven sisters	Mum died from Crohn's disease when Roger was 13 years old	Dad died from a heart attack in later life – age unknown	In-depth, psychosocial interview held in a private space outside of the participant's home.
Anna	46	Academic publishing	Married	Two adult children; one child with learning disabilities who lives at home	One younger sister and one younger brother	Mum is aged 67 and lives in supported living abroad	Dad is aged 70 and lives in a retirement community in the UK	In-depth, psychosocial interview at participant's home

(continued)

Table A2.1: Adult child participant biographical chart (continued)

Pseudonym	Age	Job	Marital status	Parental status	Siblings	Mum	Dad	Type and place of interview
Janet	40	Hairdresser	Married	Three children who all live at home	One older sister (Lisa) and one younger brother	Mum is aged 70 and lives independently without care	Dad died aged 67 from a heart attack	In-depth, psychosocial interview at participant's home
Lisa	45	Hairdresser	Married	Two adult children	One younger sister (Janet) and one younger brother	Mum is aged 70 and lives independently without care	Dad died aged 67 from a heart attack	In-depth, psychosocial interview at participant's home
Kathleen	46	Secretary	Married	Two teenaged children	One brother	Mum is aged 71 and lives independently without care	Dad is aged 73 and lives independently without care	In-depth, psychosocial interview at participant's home

Table A2.2: Older people living in care biographical chart

Pseudonym	Age	Parental status	Type and place of interview
Coral	84	One daughter	Semi-structured interview in a care home
Betty	86	No children	Semi-structured interview in a care home
Elisabeth	84	Two sons and a daughter	Semi-structured interview in a care home
Mildred	86	One son and one daughter	Semi-structured interview in a care home
Mr Randall	98	One son and one daughter	Semi-structured interview in a care home
Maeve	79	Three sons – one who had died	Semi-structured interview in a care home
Missy	90	One daughter	Semi-structured interview in a care home
Joan	87	Two daughters and one son	Semi-structured interview in a care home
Valentina	Unknown but approximately 90	Unknown	Semi-structured interview in a care home
Reverend Dawson	86	Two sons and a daughter – daughter has died	Semi-structured interview in a care home
Penelope	95	Four children – youngest daughter died	Semi-structured interview in a care home
Diana	99	One daughter (Trina)	Semi-structured interview in a care home
Joy	Unknown but approximately mid 80s	One daughter	Semi-structured interview in a care home
Martha	90	No children but two women who she 'adopted' as her own in adulthood	Semi-structured interview in a care home
Rita	Unknown but approximately mid 80s	Unknown	Semi-structured interview in a care home
Daisy	90	No children	Semi-structured interview in a care home
Jessie	Unknown but approximately mid 80s	One daughter	Semi-structured interview in a care home
Dot	Unknown but approximately mid 80s	Unknown	Observation in a care home
Jackie	Unknown but approximately mid 80s	Unknown	Observation in a care home

Table A2.3: Staff and volunteers chart

Pseudonym	Role	Type and place of interview
Rhonda	Care home manager	Semi-structured interview and observation of role in the care home
Angela	Care home manager	Semi-structured interview and observation of role in the care home
Deena	Care home manager	Semi-structured interview and observation of role in the care home
Sheila	Care home manager	Semi-structured interview and observation of role in the care home
Tina	Care home manager	Semi-structured interview and observation of role in the care home
Susan	Community volunteer	Semi-structured interview and observation of role in the care home
Veronica	Community volunteer	Semi-structured interview and observation of role in the care home
Lydia	Community volunteer	Semi-structured interview and observation of role in the care home
Ashleigh	Community volunteer	Semi-structured interview and observation of role in the care home
Anna	Community volunteer	Semi-structured interview and observation of role in the care home
Clive (aged 94)	Husband of care home resident (Joan)	Semi-structured interview and observation of role in the care home

References

Achenbaum, W. (2005) 'Ageing and changing: international historical perspectives on ageing', in M. Johnson, V. Bengtson, P. Coleman and T. Kirkwood (eds) *The Cambridge Handbook of Age and Ageing*, Cambridge: Cambridge University Press, pp 21–9.

Age UK (2019) 'You are not alone: advice and support following bereavement', [online], Available from: https://www.ageuk.org.uk/globa lassets/age-uk/documents/reports-and-publications/reports-and-briefi ngs/loneliness/you-are-not-alone-report.pdf

Age UK (2020) '81,240 reasons why the over-75s TV licence should stay free', July, [online], Available from: https://www.ageuk.org.uk/latest-press/articles/2020/07/81240-reasons-why-the-over-75s-tv-licence-sho uld-stay-free/

Age UK (2021) 'Same as it ever was: "Life during the pandemic was no different to normal … I'm always lonely": loneliness and Covid-19', December, [online], Available from: https://www.ageuk.org.uk/globa lassets/age-uk/documents/reports-and-publications/consultation-respon ses-and-submissions/health--wellbeing/loneliness-and-covid-19---decem ber-2021.pdf

Age UK (January 2022) Health and Care Bill Committee Stage Briefing (Lords). Available from: https://www.ageuk.org.uk/globalassets/age-uk/ documents/reports-and-publications/reports-and-briefings/hsc-lords-committee-stage-briefing---january-2022.pdf

Akinrolie, O., Okoh, A., and Kalu, M. (2020) 'Intergenerational support between older adults and adult children in Nigeria: the role of reciprocity', *Journal of Gerontological Social Work*, 63: 478–98.

Ambiguous Loss (2023) [online], Available from: www.ambiguousloss.com/

Amundsen, D. (2022) 'Being called "elderly" impacts adult development: a critical analysis of enduring ageism during COVID in NZ Online News Media', *Journal of Adult Development*, 29(4): 328–41.

Angell, G., Dennis, B., and Dumain, L. (1998) 'Spirituality, resilience, and narrative: coping with parental death', *The Journal of Contemporary Human Services*, 79(6): 615–30.

Arber, S., and Ginn, J. (1993) 'Class, caring and the life course', in S. Arber and M. Evandrou (eds) *Aging, Independence and the Life Course*, London: Jessica Kingsley Publishers, pp 149–68.

Arbuckle, N., and de Vries, B. (1995) 'The long-term effects of later life spousal and parental bereavement on personal functioning', *The Gerontologist*, 35(5): 637–47.

Archer, J. (1999) *The Nature of Grief*, London: Routledge.

Arora, A. (2017) 'Time to move: get up, get dressed, keep moving', NHS blog, [online], Available from: https://www.england.nhs.uk/blog/amit-arora/

Arthur, K. (2004) 'Terror of death in the wake of September 11th: is this the end of death denial?', in A. Fagan (ed) *Making Sense of Dying and Death*, Amsterdam: Rodopi.

Attig, T. (1996) *How We Grieve: Relearning the World*, New York: Oxford University Press.

Attig, T. (2004) 'Disenfranchised grief revisited: discounting hope and love', *Omega*, 49(3): 197–215.

Avers, D., Brown, M., Chui, K., Wong, R., and Lusardi, M. (2011) 'Use of the term "elderly"', *Journal of Geriatric Physical Therapy*, 34(4): 153–4.

Ball, M., Kemp, C., Hollingsworth, C., and Perkins, M. (2014) '"This is our last stop": negotiating end-of-life transitions in assisted living', *Journal of Aging Studies*, 30: 1–13.

Barnes, M. (2012) 'An ethic of care and sibling care in older age', *Families, Relationships and Societies*, 1(1): 7–23.

Barron, A., and West, E. (2017) 'The quasi-market for adult residential care in the UK: do for-profit, not-for-profit or public sector residential care and nursing homes provide better quality care?', *Social Science and Medicine*, 179: 137–46.

Bath, C. (2017) 'Ethical practice in the care of an elder: a daughter's blog', *Ethics and Social Welfare*, 11(4): 307–19.

Becker, E. (1973) *The Denial of Death*, New York: Simon & Schuster.

Bee, H.L. (1998). *Lifespan development*. Harlow: Longmans.

Benson, J. (1997) *Prime Time: A History of the Middle Aged in Twentieth-Century Britain*, London: Longman.

Bernard, L., and Guarnaccia, C. (2003) 'Two models of caregiver strain and bereavement adjustment: a comparison of husband and daughter caregivers of breast cancer hospice patients', *Gerontologist*, 43(6): 808–16.

Boss, P. (1999) *Ambiguous Loss: Learning to Live with Unresolved Grief*, Cambridge, MA: Harvard University Press.

Boss, P. (2012) 'The ambiguous loss of dementia: a relational view of complicated grief in caregivers', in M. O'Reilly-Landry (ed) *A Psychodynamic Understanding of Modern Medicine: Placing the Person at the Centre of Care*, London: Radcliffe.

Bowlby, J. (1961) 'Processes of mourning', *International Journal of Psychoanalysis*, 42: 317–40.

Bowlby, J. (1988) *A Secure Base: Parent–Child Attachment and Healthy Human Development*, New York: Basic Books.

Braun, V., and Clarke, V. (2006) 'Using thematic analysis in psychology', *Qualitative Research in Psychology*, 3(2): 77–101.

Braun, V., and Clarke, V. (2013) *Successful Qualitative Research: A Practical Guide for Beginners*, London: SAGE.

British Geriatrics Society (2020) 'End of life care in frailty: care homes', 12 May, [online], Available from: https://www.bgs.org.uk/resources/end-of-life-care-in-frailty-care-homes

Brodaty, H., and Donkin, M. (2009) 'Family caregivers of people with dementia', *Dialogues Clinical Neuroscience*, 11(2): 217–28.

Brown, J. (2006) *A Psychosocial Exploration of Love and Intimacy*, Basingstoke: Palgrave Macmillan.

Buse, C., and Twigg, J. (2014) 'Women with dementia and their handbags: negotiating identity, privacy and 'home' through material culture', *Journal of Aging Studies*, 30: 14–22.

Buse, C., and Twigg, J. (2018) 'Dressing disrupted: negotiating care through the materiality of dress in the context of dementia', *Sociology of Health and Illness*, 40(2): 340–52.

Calhoun, L., Tedeschi, R., Cann, A., and Hanks, E. (2010) 'Positive outcomes following bereavement: paths to posttraumatic growth', *Psychologica Belgica*, 50: 125–43.

The Care Collective (2020) *The Care Manifesto: The Politics of Interdependence*, London: Verso.

Care Home UK (2022) 'Care home stats: number of settings, population and workforce', [online], Available from: https://www.carehome.co.uk/advice/care-home-stats-number-of-settings-population-workforce

Care Quality Commission (2016) 'People from Black and minority ethnic communities', May, [online], Available from: https://www.cqc.org.uk/sites/default/files/20160505%20CQC_EOLC_BAME_FINAL_2.pdf

Care Quality Commission (2022) 'What we do on an inspection' [online], Available from: https://www.cqc.org.uk/about-us/how-we-do-our-job/what-we-do-inspection

Carers UK (2015) 'Valuing carers 2015: the rising value of carers' support', [online], Available from: https://www.sheffield.ac.uk/polopoly_fs/1.546409!/file/Valuing-Carers-2015.pdf

Carers UK (2022) 'Facts and figures', [online], Available from: https://www.carersuk.org/news-and-campaigns/press-releases/facts-and-figures

Carmeli, E. (2014) 'The invisibles: unpaid caregivers of the elderly', *Frontiers in Public Health*, 2(2): 91.

Centre for Ageing Better (March 2022) *The State of Ageing*, [online], Available from: https://ageing-better.org.uk/summary-state-ageing-2022

The Centre for Ageing Better (17 March 2022) Government failing to ensure a decent life for older people as pensioner poverty spirals, Available from: https://ageing-better.org.uk/news/government-failing-ensure-dec ent-life-older-people-pensioner-poverty-spirals

Chappell, N., and Penning, M. (2005) 'Family caregivers: increasing demands in the context of 21st-century globalization?' in M. Johnson, V. Bengtson, P. Coleman and T. Kirkwood (eds) *The Cambridge Handbook of Age and Ageing*, Cambridge: Cambridge University Press, pp 455–62.

Chodorow, N. (1978/1999) *The Reproduction of Mothering*, Oakland: University of California Press.

Clark, A. (2013) 'Haunted by images? Ethical moments and anxieties in visual research', *Methodological Innovations Online*, 8(2): 68–81.

Clarke, S. (2006) 'Theory and practice: psychoanalytic sociology as psycho-social studies', *Sociology*, 40(6): 1153–69.

CMA (Competition and Markets Authority) (2017) 'Care homes market study: summary of final report', 30 November, [online], Available from: https://www.gov.uk/government/publications/care-homes-mar ket-study-summary-of-final-report

Comas-Herrera, A., Zalakain, J., Lemmon, E., Henderson, D., Litwin, C., Hsu, A.T. et al (2020) 'Mortality associated with COVID-19 in care homes: international evidence', *Policy Network*, CPEC-LSE.

Comptroller and Auditor General (2021) 'The adult social care market'. England Department of Health & Social Care. Available from: https:// www.nao.org.uk/wp-content/uploads/2021/03/The-adult-social-care-market-in-England.pdf

Dementia UK (2019) 'What is dementia? What are the symptoms?', [online], Available from: https://www.dementiauk.org/understanding-dementia/ advice-andinformation/dementia-first-steps/what-is-dementia/

Denzin, N., and Lincoln, Y. (2005) 'The discipline and practice of qualitative research', in N.K. Denzin and Y.S. Lincoln (eds) *The Sage Handbook of Qualitative Research*, 3rd edn. Thousand Oaks, CA: SAGE.

D'Epinay, C.J., Cavalli, S., and Guillet, L.A. (2009–2010) 'Bereavement in very old age: impact on health and relationships of the loss of a spouse, a child, a sibling, or a close friend', *Omega*, 60(4): 301–25.

Dewar, B., and Nolan, M. (2013) 'Caring about caring: developing a model to implement compassionate relationship centred care in an older people care setting', *International Journal of Nursing Studies*, 50(9): 1247–58.

Dobson, C. (2008) 'Conducting research with people not having the capacity to consent to their participation: a practical guide for researchers', [online], Available from: http://www.ed.ac.uk/files/atoms/files/bps_guidelines_for_ conducting_research_with_people_not_having_capacity_to_consent.pdf

Doka, K.J. (1989) *Disenfranchise Grief: Recognizing Hidden Sorrow*, Washington, DC: Lexington Books.

Doka, K.J., and Aber, R. (1989) 'Psychosocial loss and grief', in K.J. Doka (ed) *Disenfranchised Grief: Recognizing Hidden Sorrow*, Lexington, MA: Lexington Books, pp 187–211.

Douglas, J. (1990–91) 'Patterns of change following parent death in midlife adults', *Omega*, 22(2): 123–37.

Dupuis, S. (2002) 'Understanding ambiguous loss in the context of dementia care: adult children's perspectives', *Journal of Gerontological Social Work*, 37(2): 93–115.

Ekerdt, D. (2018) 'Things and possessions', in S. Katz (ed) *Ageing in Everyday Life: Materialities and Embodiments*, Bristol: Bristol University Press, pp 29–44.

Elder, G.H. Jr. (1975) 'Age differentiation and the life course', *Annual Review of Sociology*, 1: 165–90.

Elder, G.H. Jr, Johnson, M.K., and Crosnoe, R. (2003) 'The emergence and development of life course theory', in J.T. Mortimer and M.J. Shanahan (eds) *Handbook of the Life Course*, Boston, MA: Springer, pp 3–19.

Erikson, E. (1950) *Childhood and Society*, New York: W.W. Norton and Company.

Erikson, E. (1963) *Childhood and Society* (2nd edn), New York: W.W. Norton and Company.

Featherstone, M., and Hepworth, M. (1989) 'Ageing and old age: reflections on the postmodern lifecourse', in B. Bytheway, T. Keil, P. Allatt and A. Bryman (eds) *Becoming and Being Old: Sociological Approaches to Later Life*, London: Sage, pp 143–57.

Fine, M., and Glendinning, C. (2005) 'Dependence, independence or interdependence? Revisiting the concepts of "care" and "dependency"', *Ageing and Society*, 25: 601–21.

Foley, N. (2022) 'Informal Carers', *House of Commons Research Briefing*, https://researchbriefings.files.parliament.uk/documents/CBP-7756/CBP-7756.pdf

Foote, C., Gavel, L., and Valentich, M. (1996) 'When mothers of adult daughters die: a new area of feminist practice', *Afillia*, 11(2): 145–63.

Foster, D. (2023) 'Adult social care funding (England) commons library research briefing', *House of Commons Library*, Available from: https://researchbriefings.files.parliament.uk/documents/CBP-7903/CBP-7903.pdf

Franklin, B. (2015) 'The end of formal adult social care. a provocation by the ILC-UK', *Centre for Later Life Funding*, [online], Available from: https://ilcuk.org.uk/the-end-of-formal-adult-social-care/

Freud, A. (1992 [1936]) *The Ego and the Mechanisms of Defence*, London: Karnac.

Freud, S. (1905) 'Three Essays on the Theory of Sexuality', in J. Strachey (ed and trans) *The Standard Edition of the Complete Psychological Works of Sigmund Freud, Vol. 7 (1901–1905): A Case of Hysteria, Three Essays on Sexuality and Other Works*, London: Hogarth Press, pp 123–246.

Freud, S. (1917) 'Mourning and melancholia', in J. Strachey (ed and trans) *The Standard Edition of the Complete Psychological Works of Sigmund Freud*, Vol. 14, London: Hogarth Press, pp 237– 59.

Freud, S. (1923) 'The Ego and the Id', in J. Strachey (ed and trans) *The Standard Edition of the Complete Psychological Works of Sigmund Freud, Vol. 19 (1923–1925): The Ego and the Id and Other Works*, London: Hogarth Press, pp 1–66.

Freud, S., and Strachey, J. (1965 [1900]) *The Interpretation of Dreams*, New York: Avon Books.

Frosh, S., and Baraitser, L. (2008) 'Psychoanalysis and psychosocial studies', *Journal for the Psychoanalysis of Culture and Society*, 13(4): 346–65.

Gambone, J. (2000) *ReFirement: A Boomer's Guide to Life after 50*, Burnsville, MN: Kirk House Publishers.

Gans, D., Silverstein, M., and Lowenstein, A. (2009) 'Do Religious children care more and provide more care for older parents? A study of filial norms and behaviors across five nations', *Journal of Comparative Family Studies*, 40(2): 187–201.

Garner, J. (2004) 'Dementia', in S. Evans and J. Garner (eds) *Talking Over the Years; A Handbook of Dynamic Psychotherapy with Older Adults*, Brunner Routledge: Hove, pp 215–30.

Giddens, A. (2001 [1991]) *Modernity and Self Identity*, Cambridge: Polity Press.

Gilleard, C., and Higgs, P. (2016) 'Connecting life span development with the sociology of the life course: a new direction', *Sociology*, 50(2): 301–15.

Gilligan, C. (1982) *In a Different Voice: Psychological Theory and Women's Development*, Cambridge, MA: Harvard University Press.

Gilligan, C. (1987) 'Moral orientation and moral development' [1987], in *Justice and Care: Essential Readings in Feminist Ethics*, New York: Taylor and Francis, pp 31–46.

Glaser, B., and Strauss, A. (1966) *Awareness of Dying*, London: Weidenfeld and Nicolson.

Glaser, B.G., and Strauss, A.L. (1968) *Time for Dying*, Chicago: Aldine.

Goffman, E. (1959) *The Presentation of Self in Everyday Life*, New York: Bantam Doubleday.

Gold, R. (1958) 'Roles in sociological fieldwork', *Social Forces*, 36: 217–23.

Gonyea, J., Paris, R., and de Saxe Zerden, L. (2008) 'Adult daughters and aging mothers: the role of guilt in the experience of caregiver burden', *Aging and Mental Health*, 12(5): 559–67.

Gov.co.uk (2022) 'Adult social care – long term support. NHS Digital', [online], Available from: https://www.ethnicity-facts-figures.service.gov.uk/health/social-care/adult-social-care-long-term-support/latest

Gugliucci, M., and Whittington, F. (2014) 'Nursing Home Living: The Complexities and Potential', *The Gerontologist*, 54(4): 718–723.

Habermas, J. (1968) *Knowledge and Human Interests*, London: Heinemann.

Hagan, R., Taylor, B., Mallett, J., Manktelow, R., and Pascal, J. (2020) 'Older people, loss, and loneliness: the troublesome nature of increased contact with adult children', *Illness, Crisis & Loss*, 28(3): 275–93.

Hall, K., Miller, R., and Millar, R. (2016) 'Public, private or neither? Analysing the publicness of health care social enterprises', *Public Management Review*, 18(4): 539–57.

Hepworth, M., and Featherstone, M. (1980) 'Changing images of middle age', in M. Johnson (ed) *Transitions in Middle and Later Life*, London: British Society of Gerontology.

Hepworth, M., and Featherstone, M. (1982) *Surviving Middle Age*, Oxford: Basil Blackwell.

Hoare, C.H. (2005) 'Erikson's general and adult developmental revisions of Freudian thought: "outward, forward, upward"', *Journal of Adult Development*, 12(1): 19–31.

Hockey, J., and James, A. (2003) *Social Identities across the Life Course*, Basingstoke: Palgrave Macmillan.

Hoggett, P. (2008) 'What's in a hyphen? Reconstructing psychosocial studies', *Psychoanalysis, Culture and Society*, 13: 379–84.

Hollway, W., and Jefferson, T. (2000) *Doing Qualitative Research Differently*, London: SAGE.

Hudson, B. (2021) 'Looking ahead: an ethical future for adult social care', in *Clients, Consumers or Citizens? The Privatisation of Adult Social Care in England*, Bristol: Policy Press, pp 91–116.

Husserl, E. (1954) *The Crisis of European Sciences and Transcendental Phenomenology*, Evanston, IL: Northwestern University Press.

Ingersoll-Dayton, B., Neal, M., Ha, J., and Hammer, L. (2003) 'Redressing inequity in parent care among siblings', *Journal of Marriage and Family*, 65(1): 201–12.

Jaques, E. (1965) 'Death and the midlife crisis', *International Journal of Psychoanalysis*, 46: 502–14.

Jung, C.G. (1930) 'The stages of life', in *Modern Man in Search of a Soul*, New York: Harvest Books, pp 109–131.

Kearl, M. (1989) *Endings: A Sociology of Death and Dying*, Oxford: Oxford University Press.

Khodyakov, D., and Carr, D. (2009) 'The Impact of late-life parental death on adult sibling relationships', *Research on Aging*, 31(5): 495–519.

King, N., Horrocks, C., and Brooks, J. (2019) *Interviews in Qualitative Research* (2nd edn), London: SAGE.

King, P. (1980) 'The life cycle as indicated by the nature of the transference in the psychonalaysis of the middle-aged and elderly', *International Journal of Psychoanalysis*, 61: 153–60.

The Kings Fund (2022) 'Overview of the health and social care workforce', [online], Available from: https://www.kingsfund.org.uk/projects/time-think-differently/trends-workforce-overview

Kittay, E. (1999) *Love's Labor: Essays on Women, Equality, and Dependency*. New York: Routledge.

Klass, D., Silverman, P., and Nickman, S. (1996) *Continuing Bonds: New Understandings of Grief*, London: Routledge.

Klein, M. (1996 [1946]) 'Notes on some schizoid mechanisms', *The Journal of Psychotherapy Practice and Research*, 5(2): 160–79.

Kohlberg, L. (1971) *From Is to Ought: How to Commit the Naturalistic Fallacy and Get Away with It in the Study of Moral Development*, New York: Academic Press.

Králová, J. (2015) 'What is social death?', *Contemporary Social Science*, 10(3): 235–48.

Lachman, M., Teshale, S., and Agrigoroaei, S. (2014) 'Midlife as a pivotal period in the life course: balancing growth and decline at the crossroads of youth and old age', *International Journal of Behavioural Development*, 39(1): 20–31.

Laing, R.D. (1961) *Self and Others*, London: Tavistock Publications.

Lambley, P. (1995) *The Middle-Aged Rebel*, Shaftsbury: Element Books.

Land, H., and Himmelweit, S. (2010) *Who Cares: Who Pays? A Report on Personalisation in Social Care*, London: Unison.

Laslett, P. (1989) *A Fresh Map of Life: The Emergence of the Third Age*, London: Weidenfeld and Nicolson.

Laslett, P. (1992) 'Is there a generational contract?' in P. Laslett and J.S. Fishkin (eds) *Justice Between Age Groups and Generations,* New Haven, CT: Yale University Press, pp 24–47.

Laslett, P. (1996) *A Fresh Map of Life* (2nd edn), London: Macmillan Press.

Levinson, D. (1978) *The Seasons of a Man's Life*, New York: Alfred A. Knopf.

Lewis, L. (2014) 'Caregivers' experiences seeking hospice care for loved ones with dementia', *Qualitative Health Research*, 24(9): 1221–31.

Lightfoot, E., and Moone, R. (2020) 'Caregiving in times of uncertainty: helping adult children of aging parents find support during the Covid-19 outbreak', *Journal of Gerontological Social Work*, 63(6–7): 542–52.

Lloyd, L. (ed) (2012) 'Introduction', in *Health and Care in Ageing Societies: A New International Approach*, Bristol: Policy Press, pp 1–10.

Lord, K., Livingston, G., Robertson, S., and Cooper, C. (2016) 'How people with dementia and their families decide about moving to a care home and support their needs: development of a decision aid, a qualitative study', *BMC Geriatrics*, 16: 68.

Maree, J.G. (2021) 'The psychosocial development theory of Erik Erikson: critical overview', *Early Child Development and Care*, 191(7–8): 1107–21.

Marks, N., Jun, H., and Song, J. (2007) 'Death of parents and adult psychological and physical well-being a prospective U.S. national study', *Journal of Family Issues*, 28(12): 1611–38.

Marshall, H. (2004) 'Mid-life loss of parents: the transition from adult child to orphan', *Ageing International*, 29(4): 351–67.

Marshall, V., and Rosenthal, C. (1982) 'Parental death: a life course marker', *Generations*, 7: 30–9.

McDaniel, J., and Clark, P. (2009) 'The new adult orphan: issues and considerations for health care professionals', *Journal of Gerontological Nursing*, 35(12): 44–9.

Menzies Lyth, I. (1960) 'Social systems as a defence against anxiety: an empirical study of the nursing service of a general hospital', *Human Relations*, 13: 95–121.

Miceli, M., and Castelfranchi, C. (2018) 'Reconsidering the differences between shame and guilt', *Europe's Journal of Psychology*, 14(3): 710–33.

Miller, K., Shoemaker, M., Willyard, J., and Addison, P. (2008) 'Providing care for elderly parents: a structurational approach to family caregiver identity', *Journal of Family Communication*, 8: 19–43.

Miyawaki, C. (2020) 'Caregiving attitudes and needs of later generation Chinese-American family caregivers of older adults', *Journal of Family Issues*, 41(12): 2377–99.

Molyneaux, V., Butchard, S., Simpson, J., and Murray, C. (2011) 'Reconsidering the term "carer": a critique of the universal adoption of the term "carer"', *Ageing and Society*, 31(3): 422–37.

Morgan Brett, B. (2011) 'The negotiation of midlife: exploring the subjective experience of ageing', PhD thesis. Archived with the British Library, [online], Available from: http://ethos.bl.uk/OrderDetails.do?did=1&uin=uk.bl.ethos.531545

Morgan Brett, B. (2018) 'Uncovering the Unconscious in psychosocial research', *SAGE Research Methods Cases*, [online], Available from: http://methods.sagepub.com/case/uncovering-the-unconscious-in-psychosocial-research

Morgan Brett, B., and Tanner, C. (2014) '"We'll meet again – don't know where, don't know when": Supporting community visiting in Essex care homes', *Joseph Rowntree Evaluation Report*, February.

Morgan Brett, B., and Tanner, C. (2017) 'Independent evaluation of the My Home Life community association friends and neighbours scheme', July.

Morgan Brett, B., and Wheeler, K. (2022) *How to Do Qualitative Interviewing*, London: SAGE.

Moss, M., and Moss, S. (1989) 'The death of a parent', in R. Kalish (ed) *Midlife Loss: Coping Strategies*, Newbury Park, CA: Sage, pp 89–114.

Moss, M., and Moss, S. (1996) 'The impact of family deaths on older people', *Bereavement Care*, 15(3): 26–7.

My Home Life England (2022a) [online], Available from: https://myhomelife.org.uk

My Home Life England (2022b) 'Guiding principles', [online], Available from: https://myhomelife.org.uk/our-guiding-principles/focussing-on-relationships/

My Home Life England (2023) 'Intergenerational linking', [online], Available from: https://myhomelife.org.uk/community-engagement/intergenerational-linking/about-us/

Naiditch, M., Triantafillou, J., Di Santo, P., Carretero, S., and Hirsch Durret, E., (2013) 'User perspective in long-term care and the role of informal carer', in K. Leichsenring et al. (eds) *Long-Term Care in Europe*, London: Palgrave Macmillan, pp 45–80.

Neugarten, B. (1974) 'Age groups in America and the rise of the young-old', *Annals of the American Society of Political and Social Science*, 415: 187–98.

NICE (2019) 'Mental wellbeing of older people in care homes: statements 1 and 2', [online], Available from: https://www.nice.org.uk/about/nice-communities/social-care/tailored-resources/mwop/knowing-the-person

Nolan, M.R., Brown, J., Davies, S., Nolan, J., and Keady, J. (2006) *The Senses Framework: Improving Care for Older People through a Relation-Centred Approach*, Getting Research into Practice Report No. 2, University of Sheffield.

Office for National Statistics (2018) 'Health state life expectancies, UK QMI – Office for National Statistics', [online], Available from: https://www.ons.gov.uk/peoplepopulationandcommunity/healthandsocialcare/healthandlifeexpectancies/methodologies/healthstatelifeexpectanciesukqmi

Office for National Statistics (2019) 'People Population and Community', [online], Available from: https://www.ons.gov.uk/peoplepopulationandcommunity/populationandmigration/populationestimates/articles/populationestimatesbyethnicgroupandreligionenglandandwales/2019

Office for National Statistics (2021a) 'National Life Tables – Life Expectancy in the UK: 2018 to 2020', [online], Available from: https://www.ons.gov.uk/peoplepopulationandcommunity/birthsdeathsandmarriages/lifeexpectancies/bulletins/nationallifetablesunitedkingdom/2018to2020

Office for National Statistics (2021b) 'Estimates of the very old, including centenarians, UK – Office for National Statistics', [online], Available from: https://www.ons.gov.uk/peoplepopulationandcommunity/birthsdeathsandmarriages/ageing/bulletins/estimatesoftheveryoldincludingcentenarians/2002to2020

Office for National Statistics (2022a) 'Estimates of the population for the UK, England and Wales, Scotland and Northern Ireland – Office for National Statistics', [online], Available from: https://www.ons.gov.uk/peoplepopulationandcommunity/populationandmigration/populationestimates/datasets/populationestimatesforukenglandandwalesscotlandandnorthernireland

Office for National Statistics (2022b) 'Voice of our ageing population: living longer lives', [online], Available from: https://www.ons.gov.uk/peoplepopulationandcommunity/birthsdeathsandmarriages/ageing/articles/voicesofourageingpopulation/livinglongerlives

Office of the Public Guardian Safeguarding Policy (2015) section 5.2, [online], Available from: https://assets.publishing.service.gov.uk/government/uploads/system/uploads/attachment_data/file/934858/SD8-Office_of-the-Public-Guardian-safeguarding-policy.pdf

Ostenweis, M., Solomon, F., and Green, M. (1984) *Bereavement: Reactions, Consequences and Care,* Washington, DC: National Academy Press.

Paoletti, I. (2002) 'Caring for older people: a gendered practice', *Discourse and Society*, 13(6): 805–17.

Parker, I. (2010) 'The place of transference in psychosocial research', *Journal of Theoretical and Philosophical Psychology*, 30(1): 17–31.

Parkes, C. (1972) *Bereavement: Studies of Grief in Adult Life*. New York: International Universities Press.

Parkes, C.M. (1975) 'Determinants of outcome following bereavement', *Omega: Journal of Death and Dying*, 6(4): 303–23.

Pearce, C., and Komaromy, C. (2021) *Narrative of Parental Death, Dying, and Bereavement: A Kind of Haunting*, London: Palgrave Macmillan.

Pearlin, L., Mullan, J., Semple, S., and Skaff, M. (1990) 'Caregiving and the stress process: an overview of concepts and their measures', *Gerontologist*, 30: 583–94.

Peters, C., Hooker, K., and Zvonkovic, A. (2006) 'Older parents' perceptions of ambivalence in relationships with their children', *Family Relations: An Interdisciplinary Journal of Applied Family Studies*, 55(5): 539–51.

Petersen, S., and Rafuls, S. (1998) 'Receiving the scepter: the generational transition and impact of parent death on adults', *Death Studies*, 22(6): 493–524.

Piercy, K.W., and Chapman, J.G. (2001) 'Adopting the caregiver role: a family legacy', *Family Relations*, 50(4): 386–93.

Pratt, C., Schmall, V., Wright, S., and Hare, J. (1987) 'The forgotten client: family caregivers to institutionalized dementia patients', in T.H. Brubaker (ed) *Aging, Health and Family*, Newbury Park, CA: SAGE, pp 197–215.

Pritchard, C. (1995) *Suicide: The Ultimate Rejection?* Buckingham: Open University Press.

Raut, S. (May 2018) 'Globalization and transformation of family care', *International Relations and Diplomacy*, 6(5): 288–97.

Ritchie, J., and Spencer, L. (1994) 'Qualitative data analysis for applied policy research', in A. Bryman and R. Burgess (eds) *Analyzing Qualitative Data*, London: Routledge, pp 172–94.

Roazen, P. (1980) 'Erik H. Erikson's America: the political implications of ego psychology', *Journal of the History of Behavioral Sciences*, 16(3): 333–41.

Roberto, K., and Jarrott, S. (2008) 'Family caregivers of older adults: a life span perspective', *Family Relations*, 57(1): 100–11.

Robinson, O., and Stell, A. (2015) 'Later life crisis: towards a holistic model', *Journal of Adult Development*, 22: 38–49.

Roper, M. (2003) 'Analysing the analysed: transference and counter-transference in the oral history encounter', *Oral History*, 31(2): 20–32.

Roseneil, S. (2006) 'The ambivalences of Angel's "arrangement": a psychosocial lens on the contemporary condition of personal life', *The Sociological Review*, 54(4): 847–69.

Roseneil, S. (2009) 'Haunting in an age of individualization', *European Societies*, 11(3): 411–30.

Roth, P. (2005) 'The depressive position', in S. Budd, and R. Rusbridger (eds) *Introducing Psychoanalysis: Essential Themes and Topics*, New York: Routledge, pp 47–58.

Rubin, H. and Rubin, I. (2012) *Qualitative Interviewing: The Art of Hearing Data* (3rd edn), Thousand Oaks, CA: SAGE.

Scharlach, A., and Fuller-Thomson, E. (1994) 'Coping strategies following the death of an elderly parent', *Journal of Gerontological Social Work*, 21(3/4): 85–100.

Seidlein, A., Buchholz, I., Buchholz, M., and Salloch, S. (2019) 'Relationships and burden: An empirical-ethical investigation of lived experience in home nursing arrangements', *Bioethics*, May 33(4): 448–56.

Sevenhuijsen, S. (1997) 'De ondragelijke lichtheid van het bestaan' in M. van den Brink (eds) *Een stuk zeep in de bad kuip. Hoe zorg tot haar recht komt*, Deventer: Kluwer, pp 43–68.

Sevenhuijsen, S. (2003) 'The place of care: the relevance of the feminist ethic of care for social policy', *Feminist Theory*, 4(2): 179–97.

Shanas, E. (1979) 'The family as a social support system in old age', *The Gerontologist*, 19(2): 169–74.

Shmotkin, D. (September 1999) 'Affective bonds of adult children with living versus deceased parents', *Psychology and Aging*, 14(3): 473–82.

Silverman, P. (1987) 'The impact of parental death on college-age women', *Psychiatric Clinics of North American*, 10(3): 387–404.

Silverstein, M., Gans, D., and Yang, F. (2006) 'Filial support to aging parents: the role of norms and needs', *Journal of Family Issues*, 27: 1068–84.

Simpson, P. (2017) 'Public spending on adult social care in England', *The Institute for Fiscal Studies*, [online] Available from: https://ifs.org.uk/publications/public-spending-adult-social-care-england

Smith, S. (1999) '"Now that mom is in The Lord's arms, i just have to live the way she taught me": reflections on an elderly, African American mother's death', *Journal of Gerontological Social Work*, 32(2): 41–51.

Spencer, L. Ritchie, J. O'Connor, W., Morrell, G and Ormston, R. (2014) 'Analysis in Practice' in Ritchie, J., Lewis, J., McNaughton Nicholls, C. and Ormston, R. *Qualitative Research Practice* (2nd Ed) London: SAGE, pp 295–345.

Spillius, E. Bott (1988) *Melanie Klein Today*, New York: Taylor and Francis.

Sprang, G., and McNeil, J. (1995) *The Many Faces of Bereavement*. New York: Brunner.

Stark, O. (1995) *Altruism and Beyond: An Economic Analysis of Transfers and Exchanges within Families and Groups* (Oscar Morgenstern Memorial Lectures), Cambridge: Cambridge University Press.

Taylor, J., and Norris, J. (1995) 'Difficulties with inevitable and expected loss', *Bereavement Care*, 14(3): 30–3.

Tronto, J.C. (1993) *Moral Boundaries: A Political Argument for an Ethic of Care*, New York and London: Routledge.

Twigg, J. (2010) 'Clothing and dementia: a neglected dimension', *Journal of Aging Studies*, 24(4): 223–30.

Twigg, J. (2013) *Fashion and Age: Dress, the Body and Later Life*, London: Bloomsbury.

Twigg, J. (2018) 'Why clothes matter: the role of dress in the everyday lives of older people', in S. Katz (ed) *Ageing in Everyday Life: Materialities and Embodiments*, Bristol: Bristol University Press, pp 181–96.

Umberson, D. (1995) 'Marriage as support or strain? Marital quality following the death of a parent', *Journal of Marriage and the Family*, 3(57): 709–7232.

Umberson, D. (2003) *Death of a Parent*, Cambridge: Cambridge University Press.

Umberson, D. (2010) *Death of a Parent: Transition to a New Adult Identity*, Cambridge: Cambridge University Press.

Umberson, D., and Chen, M. (February 1994) 'Effects of a parent's death on adult children: relationship salience and reaction to loss', *American Sociological Review*, 59(1): 152–68.

Viorst, J. (1986) *Necessary Losses*, London: Simon and Schuster.

Ward, R., Campbell, S., and Keady, J. (2014) '"Once I had money in my pocket, I was every colour under the sun": using "appearance biographies" to explore the meanings of appearance for people with dementia', *Journal of Aging Studies*, 30: 64–72.

Wenzel, K., and Poynter, D. (2014) '"I'm mother! I can take care of myself!": a contrapuntal analysis of older parents' relational talk with their adult children', *Southern Communication Journal*, 79(2): 147–70.

Westwood, S., and Daly, M. (2016) *Social Care and Older People in Home and Community Contexts: A Review of Existing Research and Evidence*, [online], Available from: https://www.gtc.ox.ac.uk/wp-content/uploads/2018/07/Report-Social-Care-and-Older-People-June-2016.pdf

Whitaker, A. (2009) 'Family involvement in the institutional eldercare context: towards a new understanding', *Journal of Aging Studies*, 23: 158–67.

Williamson, T. (2010) 'My name is not dementia', *Alzheimer's Society*, [online], Available from: https://www.yumpu.com/s/3esgJIPZFBTPGjRV

Willyard, J., Miller, K., Shoemaker, M., and Addison, P. (2008) 'Making sense of sibling responsibility for family caregiving', *Qualitative Health Research*, 18(12): 1673–86.

Woodspring, N. (2016) *Baby Boomers: Time and Ageing Bodies*, Bristol: Bristol University Press.

World Health Organisation (2023) 'Dementia'. Accessed [online]: https://www.who.int/news-room/fact-sheets/detail/dementia

Young, H., Grundy, E., and Jitlal, M. (2006) *Characteristics of Care Providers and Care Receivers Over Time*, Joseph Rowntree Foundation Report, 16 October.

Zhang, L. (2015) 'Erikson's theory of psychosocial development', in James D. Wright (ed) *International Encyclopedia of the Social & Behavioral Sciences* (2nd edn), Hong Kong: Elsevier, pp 938–46.

Index of participants

References to the appendices appear in *italic* type.

Index of subjects

References to the appendices appear in *italic* type.